Caring for
Victims of Torture

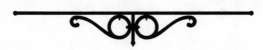

Caring for Victims of Torture

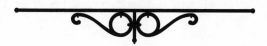

EDITED BY

James M. Jaranson, M.D., M.A., M.P.H.
Michael K. Popkin, M.D.

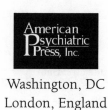

Washington, DC
London, England

Copyright © 1998 American Psychiatric Press, Inc.
ALL RIGHTS RESERVED
Manufactured in the United States of America on acid-free paper
01 00 99 98   4 3 2 1
First Edition

American Psychiatric Press, Inc.
1400 K Street, N.W., Washington, DC   20005
www.appi.org

"Devil's Island," p. vii, is reprinted by permission of the author.

Library of Congress Cataloging-in-Publication Data
 Caring for victims of torture / edited by James M. Jaranson, Michael
  K. Popkin.
     p. cm.
  Includes bibliographical references and index.
  ISBN 0-88048-774-7
  1. Torture victims—Rehabilitation.   2. Torture victims—Mental
 health.   I. Jaranson, James M., 1947- .   II. Popkin, Michael K.,
 1943- .
  [DNLM: 1. Stress Disorders, Post-Traumatic—therapy.   2. Torture—
 psychology.   3. Psychotherapy—methods.   4. Rehabilitation.   WM
 170 C277 1998]
 RC451.4.T67C37   1998
 616.85'21—dc21
 DNLM/DLC
 for Library of Congress   97-50112
                                                                          CIP

British Library Cataloguing in Publication Data
A CIP record is available from the British Library.
Cover image copyright © 1998 PhotoDisc, Inc.

In memory of Leo Eitinger, M.D., pioneer in the field of traumatic stress studies; Rudy Perpich, former Governor of Minnesota, whose vision and concern made possible the Center for Victims of Torture; and Barbara Chester, Ph.D., the Center's first director.

Devil's Island
To Sharon Olds

every time we passed the window with the poster
of a tropical paradise
sold in comfortable monthly installments
glittering with sand pink as the pink wave crests
in the wave-rich sea the rich blue depth
turned flat black and white film
even when I was only a girl and on my mind
the tropical paradise glittering with sand
became the island of my nightmares,
Dreyfus' Devil's Island.

I had often heard how they sent traitors to exile
a paradise reserved for those spared torture
the nightmare of the pink tender body its pink wave crests
trembling with the fear waves swallowing the night
a mare galloping nightmare approaching the dark eye
of the electric prod seeking the trembling flesh

the poster was my fate to be
caught in the movie theater high over the flickering lights
spreading pamphlets as the white screen flashed The End
a sad-faced girl turned traitor in a town
white mountains far away from any channel any sea
inland-locked in the terror of the times
doors slammed like iron fences clang
resounding on the silence forever in the dark

no fear for the waves the prisoners the sea
the pink-waved crests
only the geometric perfection of the fences
like Dreyfus alone in the center of the Island
fence around fence
year around year
expanding in concentric circles
over the expanding concentric waves
with the pink-crested fences
into a pink blinding concentric sky.

Silvia Divinetz, M.D.
August 1993

Contents

Section I: History and Politics

Chapter 1

Leo Eitinger, M.D.
Lars Weisæth, M.D.

Chapter 2

James M. Jaranson, M.D., M.A., M.P.H.

Section II: Identifying and Defining Sequelae

Chapter 3

Inge Genefke, M.D., D.M.Sc.h.c.
Peter Vesti, M.D.

Chapter 4

Joe Westermeyer, M.D., Ph.D.
Mark Williams, M.D.

Contributors

Federico Allodi, M.D., M.R.C.Psy.(U.K.), F.R.C.P.(C), is Associate Professor in the Department of Psychiatry, Faculty of Medicine, at the University of Toronto. Dr. Allodi received his medical education at the Madrid University in Spain and subsequently was awarded a Diploma in Psychological Medicine in England and a Diploma of Psychiatry from the University of Toronto in 1966. Dr. Allodi was a founding member of Canada's Medical Group of Amnesty International. In 1979, he was a founding member of the Canadian Centre for Victims of Torture, and he served for nearly 12 years as chair. Dr. Allodi directs the Transcultural Psychiatry Division at the University of Toronto. In 1990, he was awarded the Diploma of Recognition by the Central American Association of Families of Disappeared People.

Metin Başoğlu, M.D., Ph.D., studied medicine at the University of Hacettepe, Ankara, and qualified as specialist in psychiatry at the University of Istanbul. Dr. Basoglu settled in England and joined the Section of Experimental Psychopathology, Department of Psychiatry, at the Institute of Psychiatry in London in 1984. He is presently a senior lecturer in psychiatry and an honorary conultant psychiatrist at the Institute of Psychiatry. He is a full-time researcher in the field of anxiety disorders. Dr. Basoglu has published extensively on anxiety disorders, including panic disorder and agoraphobia, obsessive-compulsive disorder, and posttraumatic stress disorder in survivors of torture. He edited the book *Torture and Its Consequences: Current Treatment Approaches* (Cambridge University Press, 1992).

James K. Boehnlein, M.D., M.Sc., is Associate Professor of Psychiatry, Assistant Dean for Curriculum, and Director of Medical Student Education for Psychiatry at the Oregon Health Sciences University. He is also Director for Education of the Veterans Affairs Northwest Mental Illness Research, Education, and Clinical Center (MIRECC). In his clinical work at the Portland Veterans Administration Mental Health Clinic and at the

Indochinese Psychiatric Program of the Oregon Health Sciences Center, Dr. Boehnlein has treated an ethnically diverse group of trauma survivors, including Southeast Asian refugees, World War II former prisoners of war, and Vietnam veterans. His research interests include cultural factors in posttraumatic stress disorder and the impact of trauma on the family and community. Dr. Boehnlein received his M.D. from Case Western Reserve University and a master's degree in medical anthropology from the University of Pennsylvania.

Orlando J. Cartaya, M.D., was a resident in the Department of Psychiatry at Harbor-UCLA Medical Center at the time his chapter was written. He graduated from the University of Southern California at Los Angeles with a bachelor of science degree in biology and then attended the University of Southern California School of Medicine. He was an American Psychiatric Association/National Institute of Mental Health Fellow and Trainee-Consultant. He has a strong interest in minority issues as they affect the treatment of patients. He is currently in private practice in the Los Angeles area.

Lucila Edelman, M.D., is a psychiatrist and a member of Equipo Argentino de Trabajo e Investigacion Psicosocial, a team that treats and performs research concerning torture victims in Argentina. She is also on the teaching staff of the Argentine Association of Psychology and Group Psychotherapy.

Leo Eitinger, M.D. (deceased), was Professor Emeritus and former head of the Institute of Psychiatry, Medical Faculty, University of Oslo. A distinguished pioneer in the field of traumatic stress, he did his seminal work with Holocaust survivors. Dr. Eitinger received his medical education at the Masaryk University in Brno. He fled his native Czechoslovakia in 1939 but was arrested by the Germans in 1942 and sent to Auschwitz in 1943. A survivor of the Nazi concentration camps, he joined the Medical Faculty at Norway's University of Oslo and began his work examining the relationship between exposure to various stressors and psychiatric morbidity. Dr. Eitinger published more than 150 works. In 1978, he received the King Olav's Order for his contributions to the field of psychiatry and to Norway.

Inge Genefke, M.D., D.M.Sc.h.c., is Secretary-General of the International Rehabilitation Council for Torture Victims, a cofounder and an active member of the Danish Medical Group of Amnesty International, and a former president of Amnesty International's Medical Advisory Board. She is also founder of the Rehabilitation and Research Centre for Torture Victims in Copenhagen and a cofounder of the Anti-Torture Research Society. Dr. Genefke has written numerous scientific works on the physiological and psychological effects of torture. Her work in advancing human rights has been recognized with several awards, including the International Press Center's Dane of the Year Award, the Right Livelihood Honorary Award, and the Lisl and Leo Eitinger Prize.

Edvard Hauff, M.D., Ph.D., graduated from the Royal College of Surgeons in Ireland in 1975 and received certification as a specialist in psychiatry in Norway in 1983. He has served in administrative, research, and teaching positions. During the last decade, he conducted clinical and research work among refugees and immigrants, receiving his Ph.D. from the University of Oslo in 1998 for a study of Vietnamese refugees in Southeast Asia. He has also practiced as a psychiatrist in refugee camps in Southeast Asia. Since 1994 he has managed the Cambodian Mental Health Programme for the University of Oslo. Dr. Hauff is Senior Psychiatrist at the Ullevaal University Hospital in Oslo and has a part-time private practice in psychotherapy.

Karin Helweg-Larsen, M.D., Ph.D., is a Senior Research Fellow at the Danish Institute for Clinical Epidemiology, Consultant at the Danish Center of Human Rights, and a member of the Working Group on Human Rights of the Ethical Board of the Danish Medical Association. She has specialized in forensic pathology, pediatric pathology, and community medicine/public health.

Neal R. Holtan, M.D., M.P.H., F.A.C.P., graduated from the University of Iowa College of Medicine and completed a residency in internal medicine at the Hennepin County Medical Center in Minneapolis, Minnesota. He also earned a master's degree in public health from the University of Minnesota. He is a Fellow of the American College of Physicians and is certified by the American Board of Preventive Medicine. In 1980, Dr. Holtan founded the International Clinic at St. Paul–Ramsey Medical Center (Regions Hospital), and since 1987 he has served as the Medical Director at St. Paul–Ramsey County Department of Public Health. He presently holds appointments as Assistant Professor in the University of Minnesota Medical School and in the School of Public Health.

Since 1985, Dr. Holtan has served as the primary physician for the Center for Victims of Torture in Minneapolis. He has been a volunteer or consultant in Madagascar, Thailand, Uganda, and Vietnam with organizations such as the American Refugee Committee, Aid to Southeast Asia, and Minnesota International Health Volunteers.

James M. Jaranson, M.D., M.A., M.P.H., is Director of Medical Services at the Center for Victims of Torture in Minneapolis, Minnesota, and Director of the Cultural Psychiatry Training Program at the University of Minnesota. He holds a faculty appointment in the Department of Psychiatry at the University of Minnesota Medical School and founded the Internation Mental Health Program in the Psychiatry Department of St. Paul–Ramsey Medical Center (Regions Hospital) in St. Paul, Minnesota.

He is the U.S. representative on the International Council for Torture Victims, a founding member and Co-Chair of the Section on the Psychological Consequences of Torture and Persecution of the World Psychiatric Association, and a steering committee member of the Society for the Study of Psychiatry and Culture.

His academic background includes the M.D. and an M.A. in anthropology from the University of Minnesota and a master's degree in public health from Harvard University. He is board certified in public health and general preventive medicine as well as in psychiatry.

Dr. Jaranson has studied, written, and lectured on many aspects of the care of refugee patients and torture survivors. He has worked in cross-cultural mental health settings since medical school; these settings include the Indian Health Service and the regional operations of the National Institute of Mental Health. He has worked with Native Americans, Pacific Islanders, and, since 1984, refugees and torture survivors in Minnesota.

Dr. Jaranson's awards include fellowship in the American Psychiatric Association, the Community Caregiver Award by *Minnesota Physician,* and honoree in the "World of Difference" program (cosponsored by KSTP-TV and the St. Paul Pioneer Press). He has been voted an outstanding physician for the central region of the United States.

Marianne Kastrup, M.D., Ph.D., is Medical Director, Rehabilitation and Research Centre for Torture Victims in Copenhagen, Denmark. She was formerly Associate Professor in Psychiatry and Head of the Psychiatry Department at Copenhagen University Hospital, Hvidovre. She is Secretary for Finance of the World Psychiatric Association, a member of the Work Group on Human Rights of the Danish Medical Association, and member of the Advisory Board Panel on Mental Health for the World Health Organization.

Daniel Kersner, M.D., is a specialist in psychological medicine, a group psychotherapist, and a member of Equipo Argentino de Trabajo e Investigacion Psicosocial, a team involved in treatment of and research about torture victims in Argentina.

J. David Kinzie, M.D., is Professor of Psychiatry and Director of Clinical Services in the Department of Psychiatry at Oregon Health Sciences University. He graduated from LaVerne College in California, received his M.D. and did his psychiatric residency at the University of Washington in Seattle, and completed a transcultural psychiatry fellowship in Honolulu, Hawaii. Dr. Kinzie is a well-respected clinician and researcher in the field of refugee mental health and has published and presented extensively throughout the United States and internationally.

Diana Kordon, M.D., is a psychiatrist and coordinator of Equipo Argentino de Trabajo e Investigacion Psicosocial, a team that treats and performs research concerning torture victims in Argentina. She is also Professor of Psychology, Ethics, and Human Rights at the School of Psychology, University of Buenos Aires, and is on the teaching staff of the Argentine Association of Psychology and Group Psychotherapy.

Darío Lagos, M.D., is a psychiatrist and a member of Equipo Argentino de Trabajo e Investigacion Psicosocial, a team that provides treatment for and does research about torture victims in Argentina, the Argentine Psychiatrist Association, the Argentine Association of Psychology and Group Psychotherapy, and a member of the Medical Network of Amnesty International in Argentina.

Ira M. Lesser, M.D., is Associate Professor-in-Residence, Department of Psychiatry, University of California at Los Angeles School of Medicine;

and Vice-Chair for Academic Affairs, Department of Psychiatry, Harbor-UCLA Medical Center. He received his bachelor's degree in psychology from the State University of New York at Buffalo and his M.D. from the University of Pittsburgh School of Medicine in Pennsylvania. He completed his psychiatry residency at Harbor General Hospital in Torrance, California. He has published and presented extensively on biologic aspects of psychiatric disorders and pharmacologic interventions. He has most recently been coinvestigator on a number of research projects at the Research Center on the Psychobiology of Ethnicity. He has published more than 60 works and has given hundreds of presentations at academic institutions, national meetings, and community hospitals and organizations.

Paul K. Leung, M.D., is affiliated with the Oregon Health Sciences University, where he is Associate Professor of Psychiatry, Director of the Indochinese Psychiatric Program, and Acting Clinical Director of Psychiatry. He was formerly the Director of Inpatient Services and of the Psychiatric Day Hospital. He is also the Medical Director of the Chinese Mental Health Program. He received his M.D. from Virginia Commonwealth University.

Keh-Ming Lin, M.D., M.P.H., is Professor-in-Residence at the University of California at Los Angeles and Director of the National Institute of Mental Health Research Center on the Psychobiology of Ethnicity at Harbor-UCLA Medical Center. Dr. Lin is one of the foremost experts in psychopharmacological issues related to refugees and torture victims and has extensive clinical as well as research experience in this area. He has published more than 100 works and has given multiple presentations. He received his medical degree from the National Taiwan University in Taipei and his master's degree in public health from the University of Washington in Seattle. He trained in neurology and psychiatry at the National Taiwan University Hospital and at the University of Washington in Seattle. He also completed a residency in preventive medicine at the School of Public Health at the University of Washington in Seattle. He was a Robert Wood Johnson Foundation Clinical Scholar and has been a consultant for the World Health Organization and a psychiatric research mentor for minority research training in psychiatry at the American Psychiatric Association.

Ricardo Mendoza, M.D., is Associate Clinical Professor at the University of California at Los Angeles School of Medicine and Director of Psychiatric Emergency Services at Harbor-UCLA Medical Center in Torrance, California. He received a B.A. in biology from the University of Texas at Austin and completed his medical degree at the University of Texas Health Sciences Center at Dallas and his psychiatric residency at the Neuropsychiatric Institute of UCLA. He has been a Mead Johnson Fellow of the American Psychiatric Association and Teacher of the Year at Harbor-UCLA Medical Center. He is coinvestigator on research projects at the National Institute of Mental Health Research Center on the Psychobiology of Ethnicity at Harbor-UCLA Medical Center and has presented and published extensively on the use of pharmacological agents in minority, especially Hispanic, populations and in emergency psychiatry.

Aurora A. Parong, M.D., is a former political detainee. Although no warrant for her arrest was issued by the court, she was imprisoned on suspicion of treating members of the armed political opposition to the Marcos regime. She was detained from July 1982 to December 1983, 9 months of which time were spent in isolation. After detention, she joined the Medical Action Group (MAG), which renders health care services to victims of human rights violations, and served as Executive Director of MAG between 1987 and 1991. Presently, she assists victims of torture who are political detainees, former political detainees, and internal refugees. Dr. Parong is an advocate for the health care rights of all persons, as well as for the health care professional's right to render health care to anyone, independently and with freedom, even in areas of armed conflict. She also strongly believes in people's participation in decisions and actions regarding health.

Michael K. Popkin, M.D., is Chief of Psychiatry at the Hennepin County Medical Center in Minneapolis, Minnesota, and Professor of Psychiatry and Medicine at the University of Minnesota Medical School. Dr. Popkin was a member of the late Minnesota Governor Rudy Perpich's task force that advocated the development of the Center for Victims of Torture (CVT), and he served on CVT's Board of Directors from CVT's inception in 1985 to 1989. Dr. Popkin is a graduate of Princeton University and the University of Chicago Pritzker Medical School. He interned at Bellevue-New York University Hospitals and received his psychiatric training at Massachusetts General Hospital. He is past President of the Academy of Psychosomatic Medicine, has been Vice-Chair of the Delirium, Dementia and Amnestic and Other Cognitive Disorders Work Group, and has chaired the National Institute of Mental Health's Mental Health Services Research Review Committee. He reviews for more than a dozen medical journals and has written more than 120 papers and chapters on a range of topics dealing with the interface of psychiatry and medicine.

Michael W. Smith, M.D., received his bachelor of arts degree in psychology from Yale University and his medical degree from the University of Illinois at Rockford. He completed a residency in psychiatry at Harbor-UCLA Medical Center, where he was also a chief resident. As a resident he was awarded an American Psychiatric Association Minority Fellowship and a DISTA Fellowship. He currently serves as the Medical Director of the Harbor-UCLA Medical Center Adult Outpatient Psychiatric Clinic and the Novel Neuroleptic Specialty Clinic. In addition, he serves as a medical advisor to the Los Angeles County Department of Mental Health in the use of novel neuroleptics.

Dr. Smith is Assistant Professor of Psychiatry at the University of California at Los Angeles School of Medicine, where he is a Principal Investigator at the National Institute of Mental Health Research Center on the Psychobiology of Ethnicity. His primary focus in research is exploring the mechanisms involved in determining ethnic and individual variation in response to psychotropic medication.

Dr. Smith has published multiple articles, book chapters, and abstracts on ethnopsychopharmacology. He lectures extensively on this subject both nationally and internationally.

Sverre Varvin, M.D., graduated from the Faculty of Medicine, University of Bergen, Norway, in 1975 and received certification as a specialist in psychiatry in Norway in 1984. He is Research Fellow at the Psychosocial Centre for Refugees, University of Oslo, and in the private practice of psychoanalysis and psychotherapy. He is a psychoanalyst, a member of the International Psychoanalytic Association, and president of the Norwegian Psychoanalytical Society. During the last eight years he has studied and provided clinical care to refugees and immigrants.

Peter Vesti, M.D., has been a psychiatrist at the Rehabilitation and Research Centre for Torture Victims in Copenhagen for many years and has written extensively on his experiences working with the patients there. He has a special interest in the ethical issues surrounding the involvement of doctors in the process of torture.

Lars Weisæth, M.D., is Professor and Head of the Department of Military Psychiatry in the Division of Disaster Psychiatry, Oslo, Norway. Professor Weisæth completed military service (infantry) 1961–1962 and graduated from the Medical Faculty at the University of Oslo in 1968. He completed residency (1970), psychiatric training (1976), and psychoanalytic training (1984). Since 1976, Professor Weisæth has done research in the field of traumatic stress, including war, manmade and natural disasters, violence, terror, hostages, and nuclear fallout. He was a major in the United Nations Interim Force in Lebanon (1978), was a military psychiatrist (1980–1984), and has been Director of Psychiatry of the Norwegian Armed Forces and Professor of Disaster Psychiatry since 1984. He was also a World Health Organization consultant in Kuwait (1991), Serbia (1991), and Croatia (1992) and a consultant to the United Nations on compensation for Gulf War victims (1994).

Joe Westermeyer, M.D., Ph.D., worked as a general physician among refugees in Laos early in his career (1965–1967). These refugees included both people fleeing North Vietnam and internal refugees (those fleeing parts of northern and eastern Laos invaded by the North Vietnamese). During that period, he performed trauma surgery, treated nutritional and infectious disorders associated with refugee flight, and coordinated preventive programs for refugees and a rehabilitative program for amputees. In the following decade, until 1975, he returned several times to Laos after his psychiatric training. As consultant for the Ministry of Public Health and the Ministry of Social Welfare, he focused on the care of refugees with substance abuse disorders (mostly opium dependence) and disabling psychiatric disorders. In 1976, he and former colleagues from Laos established a psychiatric clinic for refugees at the University of Minnesota Hospitals and Clinics. Dr. Westermeyer is Professor of Psychiatry at the University of Minnesota and Head of Psychiatry at the Minneapolis Veterans Administration Hospital.

Mark Williams, M.D., developed an interest in transcultural psychiatry, in part through a 9-year experience of growing up in west Pakistan. He graduated from Carleton College in 1982 with a major in anthropology and sociology. After graduating from the University of Minnesota Medical School in 1986, he did a psychiatric residency at Mayo Graduate School of Medicine. During residency, he worked with Southeast Asians at a mental health clinic in Rochester, Minnesota. He then spent 2 years at the University of Oklahoma with Dr. Joe Westermeyer in a transcultural psychiatry fellowship, working primarily with Native Americans. Dr. Williams is a staff psychiatrist at St. Paul–Ramsey Medical Center (Regions Hospital) in St. Paul, Minnesota, and maintains his involvement in cultural psychiatry by directing the International Mental Health Program at St. Paul–Ramsey Medical Center (Regions Hospital) and working at the Center for Victims of Torture in Minneapolis, Minnesota.

Suzanne Witterholt, M.D., graduated from the University of Oklahoma College of Medicine, completed her residency at the University of North Carolina in Chapel Hill, and continued with a fellowship in administrative and inpatient psychiatry at North Carolina. She was on the staff of the St. Paul–Ramsey Medical Center (Regions Hospital) in St. Paul, Minnesota, working at the International Mental Health Clinic and directing a psychiatric trauma team in the Comprehensive Psychiatry Clinic. She has also worked at the Center for Victims of Torture in Minneapolis, Minnesota. She is currently a staff psychiatrist at the Anoka Regional Treatment Center, Anoka, Minnesota, where she has developed a trauma program.

Preface

The evolution of this volume is closely intertwined with the growing awareness of governmental torture and its victims. As Drs. Eitinger and Weisæth note in Chapter 1, torture has been practiced throughout human-kind's history. In many countries, this practice was and still is denied. In the 1950s, torture and its sequelae, including posttraumatic stress, received increasing attention. In the 1970s, human rights advances occurred and treatment centers for torture survivors were founded. Much has been learned about torture perpetrators and victims. The silence that has historically shrouded torture has been broken!

As the rehabilitation movement for torture survivors has grown, political forces have strongly affected the basic scientific development of the field. In Chapter 2, Dr. Jaranson describes how this tension between politics and science, and the variability in political processes, has affected research, treatment, and prevention efforts. In fact, so important is this dynamic that one can consider it the central explanatory model for the torture rehabilitation movement.

Caregivers for victims come from a myriad of backgrounds. Caregivers include medical professionals, persons from the broader field of mental health and social services, and those without formal training. Religious leaders, lawyers, politicians, human rights advocates, and torture victims are vocal in support of survivors and their needs. Often the agendas and conceptual models of these groups conflict, and there may not be unanimity within a given group. For example, psychiatrists bridge the medical and mental health domains; their possible role as psychotherapists is determined by factors such as cost and availability of therapists from other disciplines. The roles of training and education, treatment of victims, and research, as well as of public education and advocacy, are not easily blended. As a result, the focus of the field has tended to be diffuse.

Embedded in this volume are the perspectives of physicians, all of whom have worked extensively with victims of torture or have researched issues of governmental torture. This international group of contributors includes pioneers in the field of traumatic stress, such as the late Dr.

Eitinger, and founders of the earliest treatment centers, Dr. Genefke in Copenhagen and Dr. Allodi in Toronto. Drs. Jaranson, Popkin, and Holtan were involved with the 1985 founding of the first torture rehabilitation center in the United States, the Center for Victims of Torture in Minneapolis, Minnesota.

Contributors working in large, institutional medical settings include Drs. Westermeyer, Kinzie, Boehnlein, Leung, Hauff, and Varvin. Some of the authors (Drs. Holtan, Jaranson, Williams, and Witterholt) have worked with torture victims both in freestanding centers and in hospital clinics. Like Dr. Eitinger, Dr. Basoglu and Dr. Smith and colleagues are primarily researchers. Others, such as Dr. Vesti, have a special interest in ethics.

The aforementioned contributors have in common that their work is conducted in relative safety for both themselves and the survivors of torture (e.g., in countries to which victims have fled). As a counterpoint, the volume closes with the observations of physicians whose interventions have put them in harm's way. Dr. Parong and Dr. Kordon and colleagues speak from the countries in which the torture in question has been perpetrated. Other physicians, such as Dr. Mahboob Mehdi of Pakistan, were kept from being heard by repressive measures directed at their treatment efforts. We salute the remarkable courage of this special group of contributors and physicians.

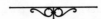

The book is divided into six sections: history and politics, identifying and defining the sequelae of torture, the role of assessment, treatment interventions, ethical implications, and voices from the field.

James M. Jaranson, M.D., M.A., M.P.H.
Michael K. Popkin, M.D.

Acknowledgments

The editors acknowledge the assistance of Sandy Rizzo, Nancy Weinzetl, and Janet Polich in the preparation of the manuscript and Steven J. Vite in copyediting. We also thank Dr. Richard C. W. Hall, who coordinated the peer review process for the book chapters, and Dr. Barbara Harrell-Bond of the Refugee Studies Programme at Oxford University for coordinating reviews of the completed manuscript; Drs. Eduardo Colón and Silvia Romero for translating and editing Chapter 12; Cheryl Robertson, R.N., M.P.H., and Garland Meadows, Ph.D., of the Center for Victims of Torture (CVT) for their comments on Chapter 14; and Libby Tata Arcel, M.A., professor of clinical psychology, University of Copenhagen, and consultant to the Rehabilitation and Research Centre for Torture Victims/International Rehabilitation Council for Torture Victims, for her work on the final draft of Chapter 3. We thank the other staff and supporters of CVT and the torture survivors treated there, without whom this book would not have been completed. Finally, the program directors from the former Yugoslavia, who participated in the training program in Minneapolis, Minnesota, were invaluable in sharing and learning with us at CVT in 1993 and 1994.

Editors' Comments

Does torture evoke a predictable constellation of signs and symptoms? Are its sequelae discrete? Do they constitute a specific syndrome? Although hardly new, these questions, the focus of Section II, continue to create controversy. One impetus for the work described in this volume was the effort by Amnesty International to document the use of torture. Torturers often seek techniques that minimize the evidence of physical sequelae. Psychic scars are often more manifest and persistent.

In recent years, the influence of North American psychiatric nosology has shifted focus away from the question of the existence of a "torture syndrome" toward the prevalence of posttraumatic stress disorder (PTSD) in survivors of torture. This shift is in response to critics such as Dr. Allodi, who decries "an ill-assorted cluster of independent 'syndromes' impossible to describe or compare according to any criteria or standards" (Chapter 5).

Consequently, politics and psychiatric diagnosis come face to face. In a matrix in which some object to medicalization or reductionism of the sociopolitical problem of torture, we offer the contrasting views of two sets of physicians. In Chapter 3, Dr. Genefke and Dr. Vesti, pioneers in the documentation of torture, detail a series of "surprises" they discovered in their work. They note that "the criteria for PTSD are not sufficient for the categorization of the entire picture after torture" (p. 50), but they contend that those who survive governmental torture can readily be identified.

If Drs. Genefke and Vesti argue for a torture syndrome, Drs. Westermeyer and Williams take a different tack. In Chapter 4, they formally compare three groups of Southeast Asian victims: those who experienced deliberate harm or threat of harm, those who experienced impersonal harm or threat of harm, and those who experienced no deliberate harm or threat of harm. They find considerable overlap and suggest that the victimized groups do not constitute a clinically unique group.

How are such opposing constructs reconciled? Is this a matter of nosology, individual differences, political and sociocultural factors, or differences in the populations studied? Most significantly, how does one gauge the contribution of torture versus the effects of the broader stressors confronting refugee populations? We note that the constructs of these two sets of clinicians have different implications for treatment (as discussed in Section IV).

In Section III, the focus is on whether there may be a special role for physicians in the work with survivors of torture. Should the physician's role be restricted to clinical care or should it encompass research, education, and policy? Physicians have been instrumental in the development of the field. However, physician complicity with torturers, as well as issues of cost and availability, have limited the physician's role. Some would argue that the medical profession brings a comprehensive perspective and the clearest appreciation of the biopsychosocial model. The psychiatrist, more than others in the mental health field, should provide expertise in mind-body issues and be versed in the psychosomatic symptoms so prevalent in victims of torture. Others would restrict the physician's role to addressing physical sequelae of torture and prescribing psychotropic medications. They would contend that psychotherapy or behavioral interventions can be conducted as effectively and more economically by nonmedical mental health care providers.

The especially sensitive issues of experimentation with and exploitation of torture victims make it difficult to conduct medical research in this field. Despite this, data addressing clinical course and outcome, with and without physician involvement, are needed. Further complicating the physician's role is the issue of power. Historically, physicians have wielded much power, but usually in institutional settings. The placement of treatment programs for victims of torture in settings removed from formal medicine has also had an impact on the physician's role.

Dr. Allodi, who strongly supports nosology and psychiatric diagnostic specificity, highlights the complexities confronting physicians who undertake the care of survivors of torture (Chapter 5). He speaks to the conceptual appreciation that the doctor working with these patients must have. Dr. Allodi goes far beyond the diagnostic manual and identifies the needed sensitivity to interpersonal issues. He emphasizes the holistic approach in which trust and the doctor-patient relationship are critical. This overrides the construct differences identified in Section II. He alerts us to the pain of retelling and the forensic tasks at hand. Dr. Holtan, an internist, notes the interplay of primary physician and psychiatrist in this work. He reminds us that the medical assessment objectifies physical sequelae, identifies medical illness presenting as psychiatric disorder, reassures the patient, and is prelude to the ongoing therapeutic, healing relationship. The medical evaluation sets the stage for ensuing psychotherapeutic treatment. Both authors discuss the physician's role in supporting requests for asylum.

In Section IV, the point is made that, although theoretical constructs abound, data regarding treatment interventions with victims of torture are very limited. Such data as are extant focus predominantly on those diagnosed with PTSD. As Dr. Smith and others comment, "To what extent the findings from the literature on PTSD can be extended to victims of torture remains unclear " (Chapter 9). The need for outcome data is unmistakable, but, at present, systematic effort has been confined to survivors meeting PTSD criteria. In the absence of unanimity regarding diagnosis and/or "syndromes," studies of treatment intervention are left in limbo. In this section, contributors advocate different approaches to treatment: psychoanalytic psychotherapy, behavioral or cognitive therapy, and psychopharmacotherapy.

Drs. Varvin and Hauff prefer psychodynamic psychotherapy. In Chapter 7, they describe torture's propensity for "splitting off" parts of the personality and impairing the individual's ability to connect with earlier "good objects and self-representations." They look to psychotherapy to "get things started again" and to put trauma in the past. Unlike many others in the field, they argue that the trauma should not be the focus of the therapist's interest. They seek to turn the "powerless victim" into an "active survivor." They acknowledge at the outset that systematic studies of psychotherapy with these patients are lacking.

Dr. Basoglu cites encouraging results from behavioral treatments for PTSD victims (Chapter 8). He, too, asks to what extent one can extrapolate from PTSD in connection with survivors of torture, stating that "no controlled studies of the efficacy of currently available treatment methods" have been reported. He infers that the positive symptoms of PTSD can be most effectively addressed by a behavioral approach, whereas cognitive therapy may be useful in the treatment of negative symptoms and for the integration of the treatment experience. However, supporting data for these purported beneficial effects of cognitive therapy are missing.

Dr. Smith and coauthors add to the chorus of uncertainty and regret (Chapter 9). Data regarding psychopharmacological interventions with

victims of torture are "severely lacking." The authors underscore the het-
erogeneity of victims of torture and the confounding variable of cognitive
deficits. They conclude by observing that "pharmacological treatment
can be successful only in the context of a healing atmosphere" and that
"no single approach by itself is adequate."

The record is all too obvious. Treatment data regarding all of these
interventions are missing. They must be collected and analyzed if the
usefulness of different approaches and of different healers is to be appreciated.

Section V is an examination of ethical concerns about torture and
the treating professions, concerns that arise not only when physicians
and other health care deliverers care for victims of torture but when they
assist torturers and the societies that allow torture. This section includes
a consideration of ethical issues at the individual as well as the sociopolitical level.

In any society, is torture ever justified? The conflict between the prag-
matic approach (i.e., utilitarianism) and the concept that certain principles are inviolable (e.g., deontology) is perhaps best expressed by Vesti
and colleagues (Chapter 11), describing the Manhattan syndrome: Is it
justifiable to torture a terrorist in order to determine the location of a
nuclear bomb the terrorist has placed in Manhattan?

How many physicians and health care practitioners have decided
that torture can, at times, be justified? How many have been coerced into
assisting torturers? Many pioneers in this field (e.g., Drs. Genefke, Vesti,
and Eitinger) believe there is never justification for participation by
health care professionals in torture. How should the world deal with
doctors and other health care workers who are found to assist torturers?

The acknowledged complicity of physicians in torture has a potential
adverse effect on the physician-patient relationship and might make it
more difficult for a victim of torture to trust a doctor. This example
prompts an important question: can one separate the political from the
medical when caring for victims of torture? If the answer is no, how does
this complexity alter treatment of torture victims? Do the countertransference reactions of clinicians to graphic torture experiences blur their
ethical boundaries?

Vesti and coauthors review the ethical foundations of the medical
profession and discuss prevention of physician complicity in torture on
three levels (Chapter 11). Prophylactic measures are aimed at education

of medical students and "doctors at risk" of assisting torturers; are directed at the development of various codes, laws, professional activities (including fact-finding missions), and public education; and include corrective actions by courts, medical associations, licensing bodies, and national or international tribunals. In Chapter 10, Dr. Boehnlein and coauthors discuss the interface between the countertransference issues and ethical principles. Physicians often experience not only the same symptoms as victims, but comparable alterations in their attitude toward others and toward the world. The authors propose six Western deontological principles that can guide the clinician and help him or her to avoid untoward effects of countertransference. In treating a patient, the ethical principles that should guide the early stages of therapy include fidelity and nonmaleficence, then beneficence, followed by autonomy and justice in the later stages of treatment. The clinician's own self-interest is needed to maintain the personal strength and balance to continue doing this work. There are always risks of either overinvolvement or emotional distancing. The issues on every level of involvement by clinicians in this field perhaps raise more questions than are answered. Both sets of authors provide a framework for ethical guidance.

The book's final section (Section VI) is a discussion of the interplay between sociopolitical context and the need to adjust individual therapeutic interventions to accommodate to these larger, more powerful forces. Torture is still occurring, or has recently been practiced, in Argentina, the Philippines, and Bosnia. The chapters in this section are only a few "voices" from a large chorus.

Many questions are raised. Must physicians and other health care workers be politically involved to be effective "in the field"? Is the logical extension that the caregiver become an activist or policy maker rather than primarily a provider of clinical services? If so, how does this change the health care provider–patient relationship? Does the clinician reveal to the patient his or her own political views? If so, where in the course of treatment? Do the usual psychotherapeutic theories and models of treatment work "in the field"? As Dr. Basoglu argues in Chapter 8, the physician's role could be to train other health care professionals or paraprofessionals in cognitive and behavioral therapies as effective psychotherapeutic interventions in those regions where primary care physicians and psychiatrists are in short supply.

Dr. Kordon and others discuss the problems of the "disappeared," or of forced disappearance, in Argentina (Chapter 12). Although the disappeared individuals suffered torture, their families became secondary victims and the focus of treatment interventions. These authors believe that the treatment of family members cannot be separated from the socially dominant forces, whether during the dictatorship or now. The authors found that they needed to revise psychoanalytical theoretical concepts such as neutrality, grief, and psychic reality. Spontaneous group models were found to be more effective than traditional individual psychotherapy sessions.

Dr. Parong of the Philippines attests that family and community as well as economic, political, cultural, and subcultural forces significantly affect treatment and rehabilitation of torture victims (Chapter 13). Treatment approaches differ for political detainees, former political detainees, and internal refugees. Nonprofessionals have a significant role in the care of torture victims. Psychiatrists and other physicians, according to Dr. Parong, need to go beyond the clinics to help prevent torture at home and abroad.

In Chapter 14, Drs. Witterholt and Jaranson, from the Center for Victims of Torture in Minnesota, discuss ways in which those from "the field" can share theoretical approaches to treatment and program development with those in "safe" countries. From experiences with projects of the United States Agency for International Development, the authors describe two approaches: 1) bringing health professionals to the United States or elsewhere for training and 2) setting up programs on site to intervene quickly with torture victims. Both approaches use a consultative model, with care provided mainly by local health care professionals or paraprofessionals.

James M. Jaranson, M.D., M.A., M.P.H.
Michael K. Popkin, M.D.

Section I

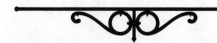

History and
Politics

CHAPTER 1

Torture
History, Treatment, and Medical Complicity

Leo Eitinger, M.D.
Lars Weisæth, M.D.

Torture has been used throughout history, and probably before a written history existed. We can read about torture in the Bible, the Second Book of Kings (25:7): "And they slew the sons of Zedekiah before his eyes and then put out the eyes of Zedekiah, and bound him in fetters, and carried him to Babylon."

This was the generally accepted way for a victorious king to deal with the defeated enemy. The main reason for this kind of mental and physical torture was to demonstrate the superiority of the former and the helplessness of the latter. This is perhaps best illustrated by the story of Basil II, under whose reign the Byzantine Empire reached its apogee. Basil succeeded in capturing 14,000 Bulgarian soldiers. These men were blinded and sent back to the Bulgarian czar Samuel in groups of 100, each group being led by one man who had had only one eye put out. When Samuel beheld the gruesome spectacle, he fell into delirium and died within 2 days. His kingdom was then annexed to the Empire (Hoefer and Goltz 1988).

But torture was not used solely for this purpose. The Church discovered early on that torture was a useful instrument for keeping the people on the right path, and it used torture on a very large scale to discourage heretics from challenging its dogma. Every person who was found guilty of religious aberration, be it as a sorcerer, a witch, or a heretic, had to expiate the crime, usually first by being tortured, then by being burned at the stake. However, it was not always so easy to determine precisely who really was guilty, and torture became a widely used method to force the suspects to tell the truth, or, rather, what the judges wanted to hear. It is only natural that such an "effective" method was adopted by other inquisitors, and third-degree interrogation became accepted more or less all over the world for many centuries. It was not until the first human rights declaration in 1789 that the idea of human dignity prevailed and torture was officially abolished, first in France and then in most countries that wanted to be considered civilized.

Denial of the Practice of Torture

In many countries not considered civilized, torture continued, and to a certain degree the same must be said of many civilized countries, where maltreatment of prisoners by flogging and other forms of cruelty was common. It is ironic—and a stigma on European civilization—that protests against torture by the clergy and physicians (by definition representatives of humanism and mercy) and members of other academic professions were few. This is a consequence of the fact that society was dominated by powerful men (the victors) and the weak (the victims) ranked low in medical and public opinion. Slowly the idea of humanism gained ground. The founding of the Red Cross in 1863 was the first international step toward helping the wounded of both sides in a war; this organization was concerned with the fate of victims only. The tortured, however, remained mute and unnoticed.

It is possible that the practice of torture had diminished by the beginning of this century. However, the blindness of the intellectuals of the pre–World War II period was so complete that they did not see, or psychologically were unable to see, what was going on in their countries and especially in the dictatorships that had sprung up after World War I. Whatever the reasons, the protests against the way political opponents were treated in the various dictatorships—Fascist Italy, the Communist Soviet Union, the dictatorships in South America—were minimal. Furthermore, the maltreatment by the colonial powers of opposing native groups fighting for freedom and independence was an accepted fact and was virtually not discussed in polite society.

The use of torture during World War II assumed such horrible dimensions and became so widely known that previous lack of interest and denial by professional groups changed to a quest for knowledge.

After World War II: Emerging Research Interest

After World War II, the situation changed in many ways. One of the reasons given often in the literature was the gruesome and heinous maltreatment to which prisoners were subjected in Nazi Germany's and Japan's prisons and camps. Many prisoners of war, who experienced the appalling treatment and deprivations in jails or in forced labor and extermination camps, were considered freedom fighters by the people to whom they returned after their sufferings. But even if they were celebrated as heroes after their return to their homelands, they had been victims and were marked physically and mentally by the wounds and scars from their experiences in captivity. They aroused the interest of the medical world in the liberated countries in Europe. The results of the research performed— both Danish and Norwegian researchers were among the leaders in this field—were unexpected and dramatic (Eitinger 1964; Eitinger and Strøm 1973). One could prove without any doubt that there were long-term stressful consequences. Even 35 years after the liberation, more survivors of the concentration camps were dying per year than predicted by demographic statistics, and the survivors examined were more often and more seriously ill than control subjects who had not been exposed to the maltreatment of the camps. Psychic disturbances during the imprisonment were more frequent in prisoners who had been exposed to very severe torture. The concentration camp syndrome was more frequent during postwar years among those who had experienced severe or very severe torture. Severity of torture also correlated with the incidence of inflicted head injuries and postwar intellectual impairment, as well as with abuse of alcohol and drugs (Strøm 1968). Torture had been used not only to force the victims to disclose their illegal activities, but also, or perhaps chiefly, to crush the psychological resistance of the arrested and thus destroy their personalities.

The more subtle but no less gruesome modern developments in torture still have these goals as their main purpose, and the evil of torture continued to plague the world in the 1960s, in the 1970s, and up through today. A recent sinister development is that some victims of torture, such as individuals and groups exposed to terrorism and political hostage, are threatened, tortured, or killed mainly as a way of exerting pressure on a third party. Not only are these victims innocent, but they usually have no connection with the political situation. Thus their torture becomes meaningless. In one case, the captors wrongly believed that the victims were secret agents. Needless to say, torture under such circumstances in peacetime has severe psychiatric consequences for many (Weisæth 1989).

Present-Day Attitudes Toward Torture

How acceptable torture has become in the minds of some of our world's leaders is demonstrated clearly by Carlos Franqui, a former close associate of the Cuban dictator Fidel Castro, in his book *Portrato de familia con Fidel (Family Portrait With Fidel)* (Franqui 1982). Franqui complains to Castro that torture has been practiced in Cuba after the revolution, and the following conversation takes place (our English translation of the Norwegian translation of the book, *Familieportrett med Fidel*):

> Castro: This is an effective method that the police use nearly all over the world and that has been used in all times. Torture is not executed by bad people. It is a practical, functional method that helps to erase the enemy.
>
> Franqui: But did you think about the moral degradation? The danger that revolutionary police or the people's army is exposed to by executing torture? You can never stop it after it has become an established norm or method.
>
> "'Yes,' Fidel says, 'it seems to be true what you are saying.

I give you my word of honor that this is an exceptional case and it will never be repeated.' And he adds, 'This revolution executes but does not torture'" (Franqui 1982).

We have many proofs showing clearly how Castro has failed to keep his word of honor. Here only two should be mentioned: Armando Valladares, who had been a prisoner in Cuba for 22 years and was tortured and maltreated in the most unbelievable ways, dedicated his book, *Against All Hope,* to the memory of his tortured and murdered comrades in Fidel Castro's prisons and to the thousands of prisoners who still suffer in these prisons (Valladares 1986). The second proof is a collection of documents and testimonies on the misuse of psychiatry on dissidents in Cuba. It is not easy for a victim of psychiatric abuse to come forward to discuss his or her experiences. These victims are to a certain degree in the same position as victims of sexual assault, in that public exposure of their humiliation usually provokes more ostracism than compassion. In this context, the documents presented and published by Brown and Lago (1989) are of importance.

For many years after World War II, torture was considered essential, indispensable, and nearly ubiquitous in time and space by dictators such as Castro; yet the contemporary characteristics of torture were not considered important enough to be studied by members of the sociomedical professions as a source of human suffering so that the victims could be helped. Public opinion did not approve or condone torture during this period, and the leaders of regimes in which torture was practiced did not want any international publicity about their methods. In the diplomatic sphere, they would deny their use of torture, but on the domestic scene they allowed rumors about its existence to flourish so that the leaders could spread fright and keep themselves in power. However, passive disapproval of torture by no means proved effective against its use, and some initiative was needed to make the civilized world take active steps against the evil.

The 1970s: Breakthrough

It was not a medical organization but a human rights organization, Amnesty International, that started the crusade against torture. The organization held a conference in December 1973 to discuss how to find evidence that torture had taken place and how to abolish the practice. Medical doctors were asked to participate in this work. Members of Amnesty International traveled often to countries where torture allegedly had taken place, and they asked doctors to provide supporting medical evidence that torture had occurred (Amnesty International 1977). The following is an excerpt (our English translation) from *Torturen i verden—den angaar oss alle* (Torture in the World: The Concern of Us All) (Genefke 1986), a history of the organization:

> We started our work in 1974. Since there were no systematic medical reports about people who had been tortured, we were obliged to investigate torture victims ourselves. We did that partly by examining Chilean refugees who lived in Denmark, partly by traveling to Greece and by examining torture victims there. The Chilean refugees in Denmark were unbelievably helpful; they understood immediately that we were trying to do something real against torture. It was obviously not easy for them to sit and talk to us about all the terrible experiences they had gone through. We got much important information from them and we can't thank them enough for the help they gave us during the difficult beginning of our work. . . . After the fall of the military junta in Greece in 1973 we could travel freely to this country. Greek colleagues helped us in talking to and examining the torture victims there. We learned quickly that though one has problems with one's body after torture, the most difficult and most important problems are of a psychic nature (Genefke 1986, pp. 14–15).

We believe this doctor's account is the beginning of the medical world's practical and theoretical concern with torture.

Usually, the first and perhaps most important step in dealing with a serious health problem is to diagnose the phenomenon and find the etiological agent. In the case of torture, the situation was somewhat different. There were people who allegedly had been tortured, but those who allegedly had executed the torture denied vehemently that the symptoms and signs found in the victims had any connection whatsoever with torture, which, according to their statements, had never taken place. Therefore, it was important to prove that the pathological signs were indeed caused by the torture applied and not by any other external (or internal) agent. It was just as important to find out whether torture had long-lasting pathogenic effects, somatic and/or psychological, and whether there could also be delayed effects, as had been found in concentration camp survivors.

At the beginning of these studies, none of these questions could be considered settled. Now, after the examination of hundreds of survivors, one can state with scientific certainty that torture causes acute and long-term somatic and, especially, psychological symptoms. It has also been possible to prove that certain pathological changes are caused mainly or only by the specific torture applied. There is reasonable hope that, with further research, more sophisticated methods of identifying symptoms of torture will be developed so that we will be able to prove the application of torture beyond any reasonable doubt.

Establishment of the Rehabilitation and Research Centre for Torture Victims in Copenhagen

Naturally enough, the next step was to ensure that tortured survivors not only were diagnosed but also were helped. It was, however, beyond the resources of Amnesty International as an organization to take on this task. The solution to the problem was found through the ingenuity and persistence of the Danish medical group attached to Amnesty International, with Inge Genefke as the driving force. After struggles with red tape and after many meetings, discussions, misunderstandings, and resolutions, this group established the first Rehabilitation and Research Centre for Torture Victims (RCT) in Copenhagen. It was not easy work, but it was extremely important and necessary, as demonstrated by RCT's role as a model for many countries, not only those accepting refugees, such as Canada, the United States, and France, but also those in which torture had been practiced earlier, such as Chile, the Philippines, Greece, and Turkey.

The work carried out by these centers has been successful in several ways. First, the survivors of torture have benefited from therapeutic interventions. Second, the treatment team has learned how highly specific and multifaceted the therapeutic approach must be. For instance, an electrocardiogram can provoke anxiety in a tortured person because it brings back memories of electric "treatment" under torture. Third, it has been learned that the therapeutic approach must be all encompassing and include somatic and psychological therapy, physiotherapy and ergotherapy, group therapy and individual conflict resolution, and sociotherapy.

A tortured refugee has lost not only his or her country and health, security and self-esteem, but also family and social contacts and his or her role in society and working life. When the reaction is a depressed state, both antidepressant drugs and psychological understanding of the depression's background will be of little importance as long as the patient has no proper place to live, no source of income, and no one who cares about him or her.

New Lessons Learned

The Danish medical team also learned a great deal about the background of torture, the way the torturers' minds work, how they must be taught to perform their role, how their humane feelings are distorted, and how their recklessness and brutality are rewarded. The different kinds of torture procedures to which the victims were exposed and the specific pathological effects torture caused were other important parts of the new knowledge collected.

Furthermore, the Danish medical team and professionals at the centers that were established learned that torture survivors are people with strong personalities, valiant and impressive in their ways, with an unrelenting and unrivaled belief in their cause. They are ready to work, to struggle, and to suffer again for human freedom, in spite of everything to which they have been exposed. In most cases, torture left its indubitable traces on body and soul, but the core of the personality, the will to continue, remained unchanged.

Participation of Medical Doctors

We should point out that the aforementioned intensive studies of torture victims also revived previously suppressed awareness that medical doctors had participated in the process of torture. As mentioned earlier, torture was used to show the victorious emperors' or dictators' "superiority" and later to extract confessions. During World War II, medical doctors in Nazi Germany and in Japanese concentration camps used torture for so-called scientific experiments (e.g., studying how long a person could be submerged in ice water or be deprived of oxygen before dying), and the Gestapo, under the supervision of medical personnel, used torture in a sadistic way, as an additional punishment for people already sentenced to death.

After World War II, many repressive and dictatorial governments continued this violation of basic human rights, using torture to extract confessions, although they can often be obtained relatively easily in less painful ways. Nevertheless, the torturers continued the maltreatment of their victims; they did not want to kill them because they knew that this would not be frightening enough. Their aim was to break the mind of the tortured and to reduce the will to resist. This is considered by the dictators of our time to be the most important result of their heinous activities as they strive to retain power and to crush any sign of opposition and resistance.

During the course of extensive medical examinations by doctors from many countries connected with the RCT program, evidence of unbelievable brutality came to light. One aspect was particularly disturbing: the extent of participation in torture by health care personnel in recent years. In spite of the Hippocratic oath, which is generally accepted, not enough emphasis has been put in modern medical training on the priority of all patients' well-being, their integrity, and the sanctity of human life. The doctors' duty is not only to heal but first of all to prevent unnecessary suffering in patients. Medical history has many examples of doctors who have forgotten these duties. Of particular notoriety were the military doctors in World War I who believed that they helped their patients by applying so-called radical therapy—a source of much unnecessary suffering.

The extent to which members of the health profession were active participants in torture was shocking (Rasmussen 1990; Stover and Nightingale 1985). The torture survivors examined by Rasmussen and his team reported that medical doctors or other health personnel were present during the administration of torture, directed the intensity, and decided when to continue or stop. Argentinian journalist Jacob Timmerman (1981) gave a vivid description. Timmerman was initially told by the prison doctor that the doctor was his friend, one who would take care of him. The doctor confided to him that he was proud of the way Timmerman withstood it all, that some people died at the hands of these torturers without a decision having been made to kill them. When this happened, it was regarded as a professional failure on the part of the doctor.

The introduction of Islamic law, or sharia, in some countries has increased the involvement of the medical profession in the execution of punishment. For instance, doctors in some countries are required to perform amputation of the right hand, without general anesthesia, in persons found guilty of theft. In other countries, the presence of a medical doctor is compulsory when a prisoner is sentenced to public flogging.

Despite the fact that torture is anathema to medical ethics and that torture and participation in torture are forbidden by several international conventions, many doctors are known to have been involved in torture activities. However, very few medical organizations have confronted their members with evidence of participation in these activities and leveled sanctions against them.

Some groups of medical doctors are especially prone to unethical practices. These doctors work for and are completely dependent on governmental authorities, especially in conditions of repression. Prison doctors are often asked to help the torturers, and forensic scientists are tempted or directed to falsify death certificates and to minimize the extent of signs and symptoms of physical (and psychological) abuse. Military doctors are put under pressure to help conceal or to maintain silence about the nefarious activities of colleagues out of loyalty to the military profession.

It is therefore a high priority to deal with such doctors at risk. The most important task is to show these individuals that their ethical responsibility is not diminished and that the international general medical and paramedical conventions on human rights and medical ethics are valid, even if the local conditions are not conducive to implementing them. Assistance and protection could be offered if the doctors were willing to work against the use of torture and other barbaric practices.

These physicians should be made aware that the medical world will consider their activities criminal, that the individuals will not be accepted at any medical conference or gathering, and that their international crimes are punishable. A special international medical tribunal could deal with physicians whose activities might be considered incompatible or irreconcilable with the basic requirements of human rights and medical ethics.

On the other hand, it must be recognized that it may be extremely difficult and dangerous for a doctor to refuse to cooperate with dictatorial authorities and regimes. Physicians may risk not only their jobs but even their freedom and life and that of their families. (We know, though, from evidence given about the Nazi doctors in German concentration camps, that those who did not want to cooperate in the maltreatment and annihilation of the prisoners were, without much ado, transferred to other positions—in most cases, however, this meant being posted to combat units at the front.) It is important that these physicians know that the international medical community is ready to assist doctors who are in danger because of their refusal to participate in torture and other unethical activities.

It is the duty of every person who wishes to help fellow human beings to take a stand against the most heinous violation of human rights—torture of defenseless people. The revelation of the shocking role that the medical profession has played in acts of torture should stir our conscience and lead us to action. It is essential, particularly for health care personnel, that the stain of physicians' participation in the administration of torture be wiped out forever.

References

Amnesty International: Evidence of Torture. Studies by the Amnesty International Danish Medical Group. London, Amnesty International Publications, 1977

Brown CJ, Lago AM: The Politics of Psychiatry in Revolutionary Cuba. New Brunswick, NJ, Transaction Publishers, 1989

Eitinger L: Concentration Camp Survivors in Norway and Israel. Oslo, Oslo University Press, 1964

Eitinger L, Strøm A: Mortality and Morbidity After Excessive Stress. New York, Humanities Press, 1973

Franqui C: Familieportrett med Fidel. Oslo, Dreier, 1982

Genefke IK: Torturen i verden—den angaar oss alle (Torture in the World: The Concern of Us All). Copenhagen, Hans Reitzels Forlag, 1986

Hoefer H, Goltz T (eds): Turkey. Singapore, APA Publications, 1988

Rasmussen OV: Medical aspects of torture: torture types and their relation to symptoms and lesions in 200 victims, followed by a description of the medical profession in relation to torture. Dan Med Bull 37 (suppl 1):1–88, 1990

Stover E, Nightingale EO (eds): The Breaking of Bodies and Minds: Torture, Psychiatric Abuse and the Health Professions. New York, WH Freeman, 1985

Strøm A (ed): Norwegian Concentration Camp Survivors. New York, Humanities Press, 1968

Timmerman J: Prisoner Without a Name, Cell Without a Number. New York, Knopf, 1981

Valladares A: Against All Hope. New York, Knopf, 1986

Weisæth L: Torture of a Norwegian ship's crew. Acta Psychiatr Scand 80 (suppl 355):63–72, 1989

CHAPTER 2

The Science and Politics of Rehabilitating Torture Survivors
An Overview

James M. Jaranson, M.D., M.A., M.P.H.

The efforts to rehabilitate survivors of government-sanctioned or politically motivated torture have been caught between competing, but sometimes complementary, scientific and political agendas. In fact, if torture rehabilitation is viewed as an area of subspecialization within health care, probably no other scientific field has been so affected by political forces. As I will demonstrate in this chapter, politics affects virtually all levels of scientific activity in torture rehabilitation—from clinical approaches to basic research—and affects both the individual and the population. Of course, there are other dichotomies in this complex and diverse field, including those between prevention and treatment perspectives and those between westernized and more traditional societies. But the tension between science and politics is of such central importance that it can serve as an organizing or explanatory model for the torture rehabilitation movement.

The interaction between science and politics has shaped and continues to shape the field. Without the political support for rehabilitation, treatment efforts would never have expanded so dramatically in recent years (Jaranson 1995). On the other hand, despite considerable progress, tension between these two forces has impeded the movement from fulfilling its potential. Many governments create barriers to effective rehabilitation. Repressive governments want to control their own people by letting it be known that the people could be tortured, but such governments deny this to the outside world for fear of international reprimand (see Chapter 1 in this volume). Within the political sphere, as well as in the scientific community, the field of torture rehabilitation remains a stepchild. Competing economic and military agendas have priority in most governments. Although the study of combat veterans, victims of domestic abuse, and survivors of natural disasters has advanced our knowledge of posttraumatic stress disorders (PTSDs), relatively little priority has been given to the study of torture survivors. In fact, until after World War II, torture was not considered important enough to study (Chapter 1), and governmental torture is difficult to study for many reasons, as will be shown in this chapter.

Using the framework of science and politics, I will attempt to explain the diversity of viewpoints about torture rehabilitation represented in the remainder of this volume. The torture rehabilitation movement is defined as the worldwide effort by health care professionals and others to care for survivors of governmental torture. It has encouraged the proliferation of centers not only to treat survivors but to conduct research, to provide training, and to heighten public awareness of torture (Jaranson 1995).

In any edited volume, the approach taken by a given contributor may vary considerably. The chapters in this volume emphasize the scientific or political perspectives or blend both points of view. Context plays a crucial role in accounting for these differences, because both the science and the politics vary significantly from country to country. The torture survivors admitted to a resettlement country, staying in refugee camps, or displaced within their own countries have been subject to varying political processes. These survivors differ by country of origin, cultural background, ethnicity, extent of social support, amount of time elapsed between the torture experience and rehabilitation, age at the time of torture, and a myriad of other factors.

In this chapter, I will provide some basic background about torture and discuss whether governmental torture can be differentiated from other trauma, studied using scientific methodologies, prevented, or treated. I will also review the expansion of the rehabilitation movement throughout the world and identify quandaries that science and politics create for physicians and other health care professionals.

Governmental Torture

Characteristics and Definitions

Politically motivated torture has been used by government officials of political persuasions to either the far right or the far left. It affects the leaders and the innocent, the strong and the weak. It is a tool used not only to extract a confession, but to control, weaken, and repress individuals, making them an example for the ethnic, religious, or political groups they represent. As such, it is a most effective weapon against democracy (Genefke 1982).

Key characteristics of governmental torture include deliberate and systematic infliction of physical or mental suffering. At least two persons, the perpetrator and the victim, are involved, and the perpetrator has complete physical control over the victim (Nightingale 1990). The torture can occur for any ostensible reason, but the real purposes are to humiliate, weaken, and destroy the personality.

The two most commonly used definitions of torture were formulated by the World Medical Association (Amnesty International 1985) and by the United Nations (1989). The World Medical Association's definition, developed in 1975, is also called the Declaration of Tokyo. It governs professional standards and ethics for physicians and states:

> For the purpose of this declaration, torture is defined as the deliberate, systematic or wanton infliction of physical or mental suffering by one or more persons acting alone or on the orders of any authority, to force another person to yield information, to make a confession, or for any other reason. (Amnesty International 1985, p. 9)

The United Nations' definition, developed at approximately the same time but revised in 1984, delineates the legal and political responsibilities of governments. It states:

For the purpose of this Convention, the term "torture" means any act by which severe pain or suffering, whether physical or mental, is intentionally inflicted on a person for such purposes as obtaining from him or a third person information or a confession, punishing him for an act he or a third person has committed or is suspected of having committed, or intimidating or coercing him or a third person for any reason based on discrimination of any kind, when such pain or suffering is inflicted by or at the instigation of or with the consent or acquiescence of a public official or other person acting in an official capacity. It does not include pain or suffering arising only from, inherent in or incidental to lawful sanctions. (United Nations 1989, p. 17)

The World Medical Association's definition is broader and does not require that the perpetrator be affiliated with a government or act officially with governmental approval. Consequently, this definition includes torture as part of domestic or ritualistic abuse, as well as in criminal activities. On the other hand, the United Nations' definition clearly limits the torture to that perpetrated, directly or indirectly, by those acting in an official capacity and appears to exclude 1) torture perpetrated by unofficial rebels or terrorists who ignore national or international mandates; 2) random violence during war; and 3) punishment allowed by national laws, even if the punishment uses techniques similar to those used by torturers. Some professionals in the torture rehabilitation field believe that this definition is too restrictive and that the definition of politically motivated torture should be broadened to include all acts of organized violence (van Willigen 1992).

Torture methods have been well documented elsewhere (Goldfeld et al. 1988; Rasmussen and Lunde 1980). The most common type of physical torture is beating, and the most common forms of mental torture are threats, humiliation, and sham executions. Torturers, whose approaches are remarkably similar throughout the world, have developed techniques that minimize identifiable physical signs of torture while prolonging the psychological aftereffects for the survivors.

Survivors of torture suffer from a range of physical complaints that correspond to the types of torture inflicted. The direct physical aftereffects are as varied as the types of torture methods used. Progress has been made in identifying the short- and long-term sequelae of specific types of torture (Rasmussen 1990; Skylv 1992). Among the more carefully studied physical sequelae are those of falanga (Rasmussen and Skylv 1993; Skylv 1993; Chapter 3 in this volume) and electrical torture (Simpson 1994). Falanga, a method of torture involving beating the soles of the feet, can be identified not only through physical examination, but also by methods including bone scintigraphy; electrical torture can be identified through physical examination and by laboratory tests to detect elevated serum creatine kinase concentrations or the presence of myoglobin in the urine. Other physical problems involve changes in physical health that occur in response to traumatic stress. Epidemiologists have found that survivors of torture or prolonged arbitrary detention are at an increased risk for infectious disease, malignancies, strokes, and heart disease (Goldman and Goldston 1985). Yet another category of physical problems is psychosomatic or psychophysiologic illness, most commonly head and back pain.

Although the physical consequences of torture can be severe, the psychological sequelae usually have the most impact on the lives of the survivors. The psychological aftereffects experienced by most survivors fall within a range of responses identified not only by those who treat survivors of governmental torture, but by health care professionals who care for victims of other forms of traumatic stress. Some survivors begin to experience psychological problems shortly after the torture, but there can be a latency period of months or even years before symptoms appear. Exhaustive studies of survivors of Nazi concentration camps confirm that debilitating psychological problems can last 40 years or more after return to normal life (Solkoff 1992). In addition, the psychological problems from which survivors suffer can change over time in response to other adverse events in their lives.

Differentiation of Governmental Torture From Other Traumatic Stressors

Professionals working in torture rehabilitation have attempted to determine whether a torture syndrome exists (see Chapter 3 in this volume) and, if such a syndrome exists, whether victims of politically motivated torture can be differentiated from those tortured or traumatized for other reasons. However, the concept of a discrete syndrome has not been validated. Other research on torture survivors, in which control or comparison groups were used, has identified posttraumatic stress and additional psychiatric sequelae but has not supported the separate existence of a torture syndrome (Basoglu et al. 1994; Chapter 4 in this volume). If such a specific syndrome could be identified, this would advance the scientific basis for the torture rehabilitation movement and would be advantageous politically. The proposed syndrome overlaps with PTSD as described by DSM-IV (American Psychiatric Association 1994) (see Appendix) but also includes other symptoms and responses. In Chapter 3 of the present work, Genefke and Vesti compare the symptoms identified by psychotherapists at the Rehabilitation and Research Centre for Torture Victims (RCT) in Copenhagen with the PTSD symptoms.

The study of the sequelae of torture has become highly political, and debate focuses on the validity of the posttraumatic stress construct. Some have argued that PTSD is culturally biased by western diagnostic systems and does not apply to trauma survivors from other parts of the world. In response, Friedman and Jaranson (1994) and others provided evidence for the universality of posttraumatic stress symptoms based on evidence that some of the psychophysiological and neurobiological alterations associated with posttraumatic stress (Giller 1990; Murburg 1994) are independent of ethnocultural factors. This evidence is greatest for the hyperarousal cluster of symptoms, especially the startle response. This does not necessarily mean that the disorder exactly as defined by the DSM-IV applies in non-Western cultures, but a final common pathway does result in many of the same symptoms. Cultural differences are more important in the expression and interpretation of these symptoms (Jaranson 1993). PTSD also remains a valid construct even though it fails to encompass all of the changes that occur after torture, including the alterations in worldview or personality described by Herman (1993) as "complex PTSD" and by Dowdall (1992) as "continuous traumatic stress syndrome."

Others have claimed that it is inappropriate to label torture survivors as medically ill when then have suffered from an essentially sociopolitical event (Chakraborty 1991). This argument is supported by the fact that posttraumatic stress symptoms are very prevalent and hence "normal" after torture. However, the fact that posttraumatic stress is common does not mean that the pathogen (torture) in society fails to cause illness.

Scientific Study of Governmental Torture

For both scientific and political reasons, use of scientific methodologies in the torture rehabilitation movement has been less prevalent than such use in related areas, such as in the study of PTSD. The torture rehabilitation movement has benefited from advancements in knowledge about and acceptance of PTSD as a valid construct in the Western world. Studies of combat veterans, victims of domestic abuse, and survivors of forms of trauma other than torture have generally used more solid scientific methodologies. Hence, the reputation of torture rehabilitation has suffered within these scientific circles.

Much of this scientific lag is due to methodological complexities of studying individual torture survivors and identifying them in population groups. Survivors may have dissociated from aspects of the torture trauma or may have amnesia for some of the events. Many survivors are reluctant to admit to their torture experiences for reasons such as lack of trust, fear of symptom exacerbation, shame, or guilt. Linguistic difficulties may further impede the development of trust. Treatment, if it occurs at all, may be delayed for years after the torture, and many torture sequelae are more difficult to identify after time has passed. Identifying survivors in the general population or even in populations at risk, such as refugee groups, is equally as difficult, for the same reasons, and significant aspects of the torture experience may not be accurately identified by a therapist or a researcher.

Clinicians tread lightly, fearful of retraumatizing patients by forcing them to divulge details of the torture experience before trust is developed or by subjecting them to tests that may resemble the torture. Even the use of structured psychiatric assessment scales may trigger symptom exacerbation. Computed tomography (CT) may remind survivors of confinement in small spaces, and electroencephalography may resemble electrical torture. Concerns about confidentiality have affected monitoring of patient progress and collection of aggregate data, especially in countries where providers and survivors are still at risk of harassment or repression. The demographic diversity of survivors in many treatment centers makes it difficult to collect large enough samples of any given group for statistical analysis, and considerable individual variation exists in the amount, type, and chronicity of torture and its sequelae.

Political machinations, professional jealousies, and differing philosophical approaches all impede scientific progress in the torture rehabilitation field. Impediments to research include professional conflicts over control of and access to data. In treatment settings, the clinical demands of caregivers may be so overwhelming that no time or energy remains for research. Even though time and money are often not available to extract clinical data from such a relatively unexplored field, clinicians may hope that eventually it will be possible. On the other hand, some clinicians still believe that their experience and treatment approaches do not require scientific validation; and for treatment outcome studies there is always the risk that some approaches will be proved less effective than assumed. The emotional or political message, after all, has worked to sustain the movement even without solid data. Gradually, however, the need for accountability of treatment results will affect the funding of torture rehabilitation.

Larger political forces have made torture difficult to study. For years, torture remained hidden by governments and ignored by the scientific community. Talking about torture was taboo for survivors, researchers, clinicians, or politicians, so the silence enshrouding torture persisted. In addition, torturers have used scientific methods developed by physicians and psychologists; therefore, scientists feared that, when the existence of torture and its techniques were revealed, torturers would learn additional methods for inflicting suffering. Governments, either repressive or democratic, have had other priorities for research dollars than the study of torture survivors. Consequently, conducting research to learn about torture survivors has been, and remains, a challenge.

However, the considerable knowledge about torture, especially the knowledge of torture sequelae and treatment methods for survivors, should not be discounted. Much of this information is shared in unpublished presentations at professional conferences or in comparisons of clinical experience rather than in the usual professional literature. Data are contained in so-called gray material (not published in the professional literature) found in documentation centers of treatment programs (e.g., Christensen and Von Cotta-Schønberg 1992).

Much more needs to be done, including studies of diagnostic and assessment techniques, of the effectiveness of treatment approaches, of neurobiological and psychopharmacological factors, and of the prevalence of torture. The science must eventually move beyond impressions, case reports, and anecdotes to incorporate more standardized measures as well as advances in neurobiology.

A number of categories of needed research have been identified. The torture rehabilitation field needs epidemiological studies. Without such studies, the rehabilitation efforts cannot be directed toward the populations at greatest risk. Even today, in many of the torture rehabilitation centers, the patient populations are not necessarily representative of torture survivors (Jaranson 1993). Selection factors to treatment must be identified for a more equitable provision of services and for advocacy of those groups who remain underserved.

The rehabilitation movement has developed monitoring approaches to clinical populations of torture survivors (e.g., Bøjholm et al. 1992) but these have not been widely accepted, partly out of fear of confidentiality breaches that might occur should databases be accessed inappropriately. Nonetheless, treatment outcome studies need the information gathered by treatment centers worldwide. Tools for outcomes research, such as culturally validated assessment instruments, are also clearly needed for this task (e.g., Mollica and Caspi-Yavin 1992; Mollica et al. 1990; Mollica et al. 1992).

Despite the fact that there is considerable documentation of torture sequelae, much remains to be done. With increasing knowledge based on recent research findings, the first step must be a systematic compilation of the information available in the published literature, in gray material, and from research in progress. Based on an up-to-date synthesis of the available information about physical and psychological sequelae of torture, protocols can be developed to assist training physicians, nonmedical health care professionals, asylum officers, immigration judges, and immigration attorneys in working with torture survivors. Cataloging the documentation of torture and setting up a mechanism to update this information regularly can make it possible to identify torture survivors and necessary research projects.

Studies of the sociocultural differences in physical and psychological sequelae of particular forms of torture need to be performed; such research should include studies of the applicability and frequency of diagnoses such as PTSD and major depression. With the increases in knowledge about the underlying biological basis for traumatic stress symptoms, it should now be possible to conduct both laboratory studies of the underlying mechanisms responsible for symptoms and psychopharmacological studies of treatment efficacy. Medical treatments need to be compared with psychotherapy and social service interventions so that the relative utility of various treatment modalities can be assessed. These and many other areas for future research can elucidate the appropriateness of our treatment approaches in caring for victims of governmental and other forms of torture.

Prevention of Governmental Torture

Prevention will be categorized according to the traditional public health concepts of primary prevention (prevention before torture has occurred), secondary prevention (early intervention with torture survivors before disability occurs), and tertiary prevention (rehabilitation of torture survivors).

Governmental torture remains prevalent despite attempts at prevention. An estimated 112 countries practice torture and ill-treatment in prisons, police stations, or detention centers, and armed opposition groups practice torture and commit other human rights abuses in another 34 countries (Amnesty International 1994a). Major populations at risk include refugees and persons displaced within their own countries. These populations at risk continue to increase, and numbers as high as 50 million or more for persons living in refugee situations have been reported (Skolnick 1995). Up to 35% may have been tortured (Baker 1992), leading to perhaps 400,000 torture survivors in the United States alone.

Basoglu (1993) has suggested that short-term and long-term strategies be attempted. Short-term primary prevention efforts include educating the general public and health care professionals about torture and exerting pressure on governments to accept and implement the international conventions prohibiting torture (see Chapter 11 of the present work). Given the significant problem of members of the medical profession assisting in torture, particular education efforts have been directed toward physicians through professional associations and licensing bodies. Such efforts are discussed in depth in Chapters 1 and 11 in this volume. Education of the public is best done through the media. Pressure on governments can be applied through traditional letter-writing campaigns on behalf of individuals, such as the campaigns of Amnesty International, or through the United Nations or other diplomatic channels, to influence governments to stop condoning torture and to start paying for rehabilitating torture survivors.

The ability to participate in legal proceedings or other public means of holding perpetrators accountable not only provides comfort for some survivors, but also may act as a deterrent to torture. The United Nations Convention Against Torture and Other Cruel, Inhuman or Degrading Treatment or Punishment (United Nations 1989) states that victims of torture shall obtain redress, compensation, and rehabilitation from the state (Article 14). Those victims from countries that have ratified the convention may complain to the United Nations Committee Against Torture if the state fails to fulfill its obligation to provide financial compensation. In the United States, survivors who were tortured in foreign countries have been able to sue their torturers for compensation in United States courts under the Torture Victim Protection Act (Public Law 102-256, 106 Stat. 73, 1992).

The ultimate goal of the torture rehabilitation movement is to influence world opinion in order to stop governments from practicing or from supporting the practice of torture. Governmental torture has been exposed but still continues, and the goal of eradicating torture still appears far away.

Effectiveness of Treatment of Survivors

Treatment approaches reflect the individual clinician's experiences with torture victims, as well as professional or societal biases. Most professionals have used the knowledge and experience acquired from the treatment of survivors traumatized in a nonpolitical context and have then adapted treatment modalities to the special needs of the governmental torture survivors they help. Accurate identification and diagnosis of these sequelae dictate the appropriate care for torture survivors, whatever their demographic background and personal experiences. Treatment of torture survivors ideally involves a multidisciplinary approach (Bøjholm and Vesti 1992; Garcia-Peltoniemi and Jaranson 1989; Ortmann et al. 1987), because the sequelae of torture are acute and chronic and may include physical, psychological, cognitive, and sociopolitical problems. The approaches are many, little consensus exists, and treatment effectiveness has not been scientifically validated by treatment outcome studies.

The context in which victims have suffered and then in which they receive help partially determines their perception of both the torture experience and the treatment intervention. Treatment of torture survivors occurs in their countries of origin as well as in countries of initial and final resettlement. Allodi (1991) defined two geographic categories of treatment settings: "the North" and "the South." Countries of final resettlement, such as the industrialized nations in the continents of Europe, North America, and Australia, fall into the former category, whereas totalitarian developing countries where torture is practiced and countries of initial refuge or resettlement compose the latter. Most of the chapters in the present work have been written by professionals from the North, and the chapters by Allodi (Chapter 5) and Holtan (Chapter 6) lay the groundwork for assessment and treatment from the perspective of the Northern countries. The two chapters contributed by representatives of the Southern countries are the chapters by Kordon et al. (Chapter 12) and Parong (Chapter 13). Treatment in refugee camps, the usual context for torture victims in countries of initial resettlement, has generally been complicated by extreme lack of resources to help vast numbers of acutely traumatized survivors who may remain for an indeterminate period (see Chapter 14).

Allodi (1991) stated that torture in the North is viewed as having the medical and psychological consequences of traumatic stress and that in the South it is viewed as a component of the sociopolitical process requiring preventive action and social change. The chosen philosophical stance dictates the approach to assessment and treatment. One commonality of the two approaches is the goal of empowerment, either of the individual or of the society. A medical-psychological treatment approach empowers the individual, whereas empowerment of the larger society or community has more explicit goals of reintegrating the individual into the political process as evidence of healing and documenting the torture to expose the perpetrators.

The primary treatment for torture survivors, at least in the countries of final resettlement, has been psychotherapy (Chester and Jaranson 1994). Two of the psychotherapeutic techniques are discussed in separate chapters of the present volume: cognitive-behavioral treatment (Chapter 8) and insight-oriented approaches such as psychodynamic psychotherapy (Chapters 5 and 7). Other approaches include supportive, desensitization, family, group, play, psychosocial, and testimony therapies (Vesti and Kastrup 1992). Working with the families of the "disappeared" is discussed in detail in the chapter by Kordon et al. (Chapter 12). Newer techniques include eye movement desensitization and reprocessing, described by Shapiro (1995).

Retelling the trauma story for reframing and reworking has been a central tenet in treatment (Mollica 1988), but recovering memories of the torture must be done in a safe setting and with appropriate timing. If done within a therapeutic setting, this can lead to anxiety reduction and cognitive change. Cultural factors are also noted to be important in the interpretation of the torture experience for the survivor and in the way the symptoms manifest themselves. Treatment in countries in the South often involves fewer classic psychotherapy techniques and relies on a more community-based intervention, heavily influenced by issues such as the political climate and safety (Parong et al. 1992).

The conceptual basis for pharmacotherapy and the literature supporting treatment with psychotherapeutic agents are reviewed by Smith et al. in this volume (Chapter 9). Lin et al. (1993), in a comprehensive review, focused on the psychobiological basis for ethnicity and its implications for pharmacotherapy; and in a concise review, Jaranson (1991) discussed pharmacotherapy for refugees and suggested clinical guidelines. Centers that exclusively treat torture victims often discourage the use of pharmacotherapy, but hospital- and clinic-based programs more frequently use pharmacotherapy for symptom reduction. Tricyclic antidepressants are the most studied agents, but many clinicians prefer using the selective serotonin reuptake inhibitors (SSRIs). However, the data from the relatively few recent studies of SSRIs are inconclusive, and these studies have not been conducted with torture survivors. Psychotropic agents from virtually all of the major categories have been used to treat torture survivors. Aside from biological response differences, cultural factors also influence the effectiveness of psychopharmacological therapy and affect medication compliance.

Primary care medicine (Chester and Holtan 1992), nursing (Jacobsen and Vesti 1989), and physiotherapy (Prip et al. 1994) are important in the care of torture survivors, at least in the Northern or resettlement countries. Social service needs for most torture survivors are critical. Even in countries of final resettlement, victims often require help with housing, finances, or asylum applications. Unless the survivor has some of these social service needs met, the healing cannot proceed effectively.

In countries where torture is still practiced, the resources are usually limited. Psychologists or psychiatrists may be a rarity, or concepts such as mental health may not be understood or accepted, but the relatively more concrete help of medicines, practitioners, and social services is more easily accepted.

How can governmental torture be treated effectively? It depends on whom you ask. How does one proceed to start a treatment program? This, too, depends on whom you ask. At this point in the evolution of the torture rehabilitation movement, the responses largely are political rather than scientific.

Expansion of the Rehabilitation Movement

The definition of a torture rehabilitation center remains controversial. Differences are found in the populations of torture survivors accepted into treatment, the treatment setting, and the resources available for treatment. More comprehensive assessment of the torture rehabilitation movement can be found elsewhere in the literature (Jaranson 1995). The following section will highlight key points only.

Some centers treat survivors of politically motivated torture exclusively. Some of those centers further restrict care to persons who are legal refugees or immigrants, claiming that asylum seekers and others who lack the assurance of safety would not benefit from treatment. Some centers adhere to the definitions of torture described earlier in this chapter. Some restrict treatment to members of a particular political group, usually their own. Some focus on secondary victims, such as family members of the disappeared (see Chapter 12 in this volume) or individuals who have witnessed the torture of others. Other organizations have a broader mission, such as treating all political refugees, victims of other causes of psychological trauma, or specific ethnic groups likely to have been traumatized. How does an organization qualify as a torture treatment center—through self-definition or through affiliation with professional or political organizations for torture rehabilitation? Can a single professional be considered a center? If not, how many persons are necessary for qualification? Without unanimity in the answers to these questions, describing the rehabilitation movement becomes difficult.

Westermeyer and Lam (1989) compared the advantages and disadvantages of setting up a center that treats victims of governmental torture exclusively. Their arguments supporting the exclusive model include the abilities to raise money, to mobilize public opinion through the media, and to advocate politically. Their arguments against this model include duplication of services already available, alleged inability to provide the broad range of services needed for torture survivors, and prolongation of the victim status by identifying torture survivors as victims.

Whether treatment should be offered in a clinical setting, such as a hospital or an outpatient clinic, or in a more neutral environment remains controversial. The former model has been frequently adopted both in the United States and in Europe (van Willigen 1992; Jaranson 1993). Many of the rehabilitation centers treating torture survivors exclusively have adopted the latter model, including RCT in Copenhagen (see Chapter 3 in the present work) and the Center for Victims of Torture (CVT) in Minneapolis, Minnesota (see Chapter 14). They fear that patients whose torture involved complicity by physicians will refuse to accept treatment or will be retraumatized in a hospital or clinic.

The resources available to treat torture survivors are generally scarce, vary enormously in different parts of the world, yet influence the treatment provided. Governments may be unwilling or unable to provide financial support or reimbursement for treatment. Even in the relatively richer countries, public and private resources to set up separate treatment centers or to establish the ideal multidisciplinary model may be limited (Holtan and Robertson 1992). Some centers in the South refuse to accept money from governments perceived as condoning torture or collaborating with torturers. Professional resources may be limited by their availability or interest in doing this work. Some centers with scarce resources depend heavily on volunteers, not all of them professionally trained. In the Southern countries and in refugee camps, resources are usually very scarce. Some of the more established centers have entered the third generation and reached out to help establish programs and train staff in Southern countries and in refugee camps (see Chapter 14 in this work).

Beginning in the 1970s, the torture rehabilitation movement had its most visible development in countries of final resettlement for refugees. Because of the repressive nature of regimes in the South, much of the human rights activism and many of the early treatment efforts, scientific studies, and attempts to disseminate information remained covert for fear of retaliation. Treatment in countries that practice torture has been difficult and sometimes impossible. In South America, for example, a number of centers were started in the 1970s and 1980s, as early as the centers were begun in the North, but did not seek the visibility of many of the Northern centers. Cienfuegos and Monelli (1983) provided one of the earliest examples of these difficulties. In publishing their results using the testimony method to treat those persecuted by the military government in Chile, these psychologists used pseudonyms and disguised their mental health program.

In the early to mid-1980s, some of the earliest centers in resettlement countries were RCT in Copenhagen, often cited as the first, and two centers in North America, the Canadian Centre for Victims of Torture in Canada (Toronto) and CVT in the United States (Minneapolis). Representatives from all three centers have contributed chapters to this volume.

Since the establishment of these and other early centers, the torture rehabilitation movement has expanded dramatically worldwide. Amnesty International (1994b) identified more than 100 groups working with victims of political or other forms of organized violence in more than 25 countries. The International Rehabilitation Council for Torture Victims (IRCT) has provided training or financial support to many new and existing centers and has helped establish at least 99 centers in 49 countries. IRCT estimated there were 183 centers in 1995 and predicted there would be 296 centers by 1998. Most of this growth is in the Southern countries. In 1995 the Northern countries had 87 centers and the South had 96, and IRCT predicted there would be 95 centers in the North and 201 in the South by 1998 (United Nations 1996). However, because the definition of a center remains controversial, these numbers must be evaluated carefully.

IRCT estimated the average total cost of rehabilitation centers to be approximately $500,000 for centers in the North and approximately $150,000 in the South. Perhaps 80% of the financial support for centers in the North comes from a variety of local sources, including private foundations, individuals, and governments, and the remaining 20% comes from international sources. However, the majority of the international funds support rehabilitation activities in the South. International funds included slightly more than $15 million from the United Nations Voluntary Fund for Victims of Torture, the Commission of the European Union, and bilateral and private sources in 1996 (United Nations 1996). The estimated need for international funding in 1996, however, was more than $26 million, and it is projected to be nearly $40 million by 1998. Because the resources fall short of projected need, some efforts have been made to remedy this situation by increasing funding by international bodies. Some individual countries have also attempted to help. For example, in the United States, the Comprehensive Torture Victims Relief Act, first introduced in the U.S. Congress (S. 2362) in 1994, was reintroduced most recently on February 4, 1998, as the Torture Victims Relief Act (S. 1606 and H.R. 3161). Among other mandates, the act would authorize financial support for treatment centers both domestically and internationally and increase the contribution of the United States to the United Nations Voluntary Fund for Torture Victims. Another version, the Survivors of Torture Support Act (S. 1603), prohibits courts from reviewing the regulations issued under this law and fails to protect certain aliens who have committed crimes in the United States.

Dilemmas for Physicians and Other Health Care Professionals

The difficulties for health care professionals caring for survivors of torture are many, and a few of these will be briefly discussed in this chapter.

The burden of physician complicity with torture or severe and unusual punishment is discussed at length elsewhere in this book (Chapters 1 and 11). For doctors "at risk," such as prison doctors, or for practitioners in countries of repression, the pressure to assist torturers can be overwhelming. For the practitioner in resettlement countries, survivors whose torturers were assisted by doctors may not be willing to share necessary information. A related dilemma results: how and in what cases should doctors guilty of complicity be punished? If a doctor is to be punished, who should be responsible for meting out the justice? Should it be other doctors or some impartial party?

Confidentiality for torture survivors is necessary for development of trust and for the treatment process to proceed. When the number of survivors in treatment centers is small, it is often difficult to disguise their cases for education and media activities, which are important for the visibility of the rehabilitation movement. In counties of repression, confidentiality seldom can be assured—treatment records and databases can be accessed by governments wanting to use the information to continue the repression. What is the role of the caregiver and how does the caregiver balance these competing needs or pressures? In Turkey, for example, the government has prosecuted representatives of the Human Rights Foundation of Turkey for refusing to provide the names and addresses of torture survivors treated at its centers (Munoz 1996).

A significant role for many torture rehabilitation centers has been to assist torture survivors with applications for asylum (see Chapter 5 in the present work). Guides to assist health care professionals in detecting physical and psychological evidence of torture have been published (Physicians for Human Rights 1991; Randall and Lutz 1991). Accurate assessment of the veracity of the survivor's story is obviously important, both for the treatment professionals and for immigration officials who grant asylum. However, some professionals in the field firmly believe that the role of advocate for asylum seekers and the role of treatment provider are potentially conflicting. One of the reasons given is the fear that stories of torture will be fabricated to enable the individual to gain asylum. Other professionals question the accuracy of torture histories, citing the controversy over the implanting of false memories in patients by therapists in other settings.

Determining appropriate personal boundaries becomes a major issue in caring for torture survivors (see Chapter 10 in this book). Does the health care professional become personally involved in political action, human rights, or social change? Does such involvement interfere with therapeutic relationships with torture survivors? What effect does this have on professional objectivity?

Torture survivors' experiences predictably evoke strong emotional reactions in health care professionals, lawyers, researchers, administrators, clerical staff, and volunteers. Caregivers may respond to the survivor with disbelief or cynicism regarding the veracity of the victim's story. Other responses include suffering from some of the symptoms that torture survivors experience. Conceptual explanations of this process include burnout, countertransference, and "vicarious traumatization" (McCann and Pearlman 1990). Burnout attributes the response predominantly to the external stressors, countertransference to the internal dynamics of the caregiver, and vicarious traumatization to both factors. In Chapter 10 of the present work, Boehnlein et al. elaborate on the concept of vicarious traumatization and raise a number of ethical issues that therapists encounter when dealing with their own countertransference to torture survivors. Coping strategies include balancing personal and professional lives, respecting personal boundaries, developing realistic expectations, and becoming involved in social and political change. Fortunately, the need to care for the caregivers has resulted in formal training and support within the rehabilitation networks.

Conclusion

Politics has affected virtually every aspect of the science involved in rehabilitating survivors of government-sanctioned torture. Diagnosis, assessment, treatment, and the development of centers to care for survivors have all been molded, to a greater or lesser extent, by political forces. In the interaction with torture survivors, the philosophies, ethics, and approaches of individual physicians and other health care professionals reflect the political context. Politics has impeded the progress of scientific study in the torture rehabilitation movement, but if it were not for politics, there would be no movement. On a more cynical note, if it were not for politics there would be no government-sanctioned torture. Science and politics can never be completely separated in torture rehabilitation, and they are not entirely comfortable bedfellows. Science requires research, politics requires activism—sometimes they are compatible, sometimes they are not.

In spite of it all, scientific and political progress has been made in torture rehabilitation. Torture techniques and sequelae have been identified and can help torture survivors make stronger cases to receive political asylum in resettlement countries. Treatment centers have proliferated worldwide, and the politicians have provided funding for rehabilitation, although little for scientific research. Education of politicians, bureaucrats, health care professionals, lawyers, police officers, and the general public has increased support for the rehabilitation movement. The science still has far to go and many obstacles to overcome to use methodologies that the scientific community accepts, but there is some evidence of progress. Questions are now being asked about what was previously accepted as fact. For example, does treatment work, and, if it does, which modalities are particularly effective? How is governmental torture different from other torture and trauma? How prevalent is torture and what groups are at the greatest risk? How can we best prevent or eradicate torture? How can health care professionals juggle the demands of caring for survivors in an ethical fashion and with the tasks of conducting scientific research? We have more questions than answers in torture rehabilitation, but with the aid of science (and politics) we can learn to formulate the right questions and continue to struggle to find answers.

APPENDIX

Diagnostic Criteria for Posttraumatic Stress Disorder (PTSD)

A. The person has been exposed to a traumatic event in which both of the following were present:

    (1) the person experienced, witnessed, or was confronted with an event or events that involved actual or threatened death or serious injury, or a threat to the physical integrity of self or others

    (2) the person's response involved intense fear, helplessness, or horror. Note: In children, this may be expressed instead by disorganized or agitated behavior

B. The traumatic event is persistently reexperienced in one (or more) of the following ways:

    (1) recurrent and intrusive distressing recollections of the event, including images, thoughts, or perceptions. Note: In young children, repetitive play may occur in which themes or aspects of the trauma are expressed.

    (2) recurrent distressing dreams of the event. Note: In children, there may be frightening dreams without recognizable content.

    (3) acting or feeling as if the traumatic event were recurring (includes a sense of reliving the experience, illusions, hallucinations, and dissociative flashback episodes, including those that occur on awakening or when intoxicated). Note: In young children, trauma-specific reenactment may occur.

(4)　intense psychological distress at exposure to internal or external cues that symbolize or resemble an aspect of the traumatic event

(5)　physiological reactivity on exposure to internal or external cues that symbolize or resemble an aspect of the traumatic event

C.　Persistent avoidance of stimuli associated with the trauma and numbing of general responsiveness (not present before the trauma), as indicated by three (or more) of the following:

(1)　efforts to avoid thoughts, feelings, or conversations associated with the trauma

(2)　efforts to avoid activities, places, or people that arouse recollections of the trauma

(3)　inability to recall an important aspect of the trauma

(4)　markedly diminished interest or participation in significant activities

(5)　feeling of detachment or estrangement from others

(6)　restricted range of affect (e.g., unable to have loving feelings)

(7)　sense of a foreshortened future (e.g., does not expect to have a career, marriage, children, or a normal life span)

D.　Persistent symptoms of increased arousal (not present before the trauma), as indicated by two (or more) of the following:

(1)　difficulty falling or staying asleep

(2)　irritability or outbursts of anger

(3)　difficulty concentrating

(4)　hypervigilance

(5)　exaggerated startle response

E.　Duration of the disturbance (symptoms in Criteria B, C, and D) is more than 1 month.

F.　The disturbance causes clinically significant distress or impairment in social, occupational, or other important areas of functioning.

Specify if:

　Acute:　if duration of symptoms is less than 3 months

　Chronic:　if duration of symptoms is 3 months or more

Specify if:
With Delayed Onset: if onset of symptoms is at least 6 months after the stressor

---

Source. Reprinted from American Psychiatric Association: *Diagnostic and Statistical Manual of Mental Disorders,* 4th Edition. Washington, DC, American Psychiatric Association, 1994. Copyright 1994 American Psychiatric Association. Used with permission.

References

Allodi FA: Terrorism and torture, in Environment and Psychopathology. Edited by Ghadirian AMA, Lehmann HE. New York, Springer, 1991

American Psychiatric Association: Diagnostic and Statistical Manual of Mental Disorders, 4th Edition. Washington, DC, American Psychiatric Association, 1994, pp 427–429

Amnesty International: Declaration of Tokyo, World Medical Association, in Ethical Codes and Declarations Relevant to the Health Professions, 2nd Edition. London, Amnesty International Secretariat, 1985, pp 9–10

Amnesty International: Amnesty International Annual Report. London, Amnesty International Secretariat, 1994a

Amnesty International: Preliminary Survey of Medical and Psychosocial Services for Victims of Human Rights Violations. London, Amnesty International Secretariat, 1994b

Baker R: Psychosocial consequences for tortured refugees seeking asylum and refugee status in Europe, in Torture and Its Consequences: Current Treatment Approaches. Edited by Basoglu M. New York, Cambridge University Press, 1992, pp 83–101

Basoglu M: Prevention of torture and care of survivors: an integrated approach. JAMA 270:606–611, 1993

Basoglu M, Paker M, Özmen E, et al: Factors related to long-term traumatic stress responses in survivors of torture in Turkey. JAMA 272:357–363, 1994

Bøjholm S, Vesti P: Multidisciplinary approach in the treatment of torture survivors, in Torture and Its Consequences: Current Treatment Approaches. Edited by Basoglu M. New York, Cambridge University Press, 1992, pp 299–309.

Bøjholm S, Foldspang A, Juhler M, et al: Monitoring the health and rehabilitation of torture survivors. Copenhagen, Rehabilitation and Research Centre for Torture Victims, 1992

Chakraborty A: Culture, colonialism, and psychiatry. Lancet 337:1204–1207, 1991

Chester B, Holtan N: Working with refugee survivors of torture. Special issue: Cross-cultural medicine—a decade later. West J Med 157:301–304, 1992

Chester B, Jaranson J: The context of survival and destruction: conducting psychotherapy with survivors of torture. National Center for Post Traumatic Stress Disorder Clinical Newsletter 4:17–20, 1994

Christensen MS, Von Cotta-Schønberg M: The documentation centre at the International Rehabilitation and Research Centre for Torture Victims. Paper presented at conference, Health Situation of Refugees and Victims of Organized Violence, Netherlands Ministry of Welfare, Health and Cultural Affairs, Rijswijk, The Netherlands, 1992

Cienfuegos AJ, Monelli C: The testimony of political repression as a therapeutic instrument. Am J Orthopsychiatry 53:43–51, 1983

Dowdall T: Torture and the helping profession in South Africa, in Torture and Its Consequences: Current Treatment Approaches. Edited by Basoglu M. New York, Cambridge University Press, 1992, pp 452–471

Friedman M, Jaranson J: The applicability of the posttraumatic concept to refugees, in Amidst Peril and Pain: The Mental Health and Wellbeing of the World's Refugees. Edited by Marsella T, Bornemann T, Ekblad S, et al. Washington, DC, American Psychological Association, 1994, pp 207–227

Garcia-Peltoniemi RE, Jaranson J: A multidisciplinary approach to the treatment of torture victims. Abstract of paper presented at the 2nd International Conference of Centres, Institutions and Individuals Concerned With the Care of Victims of Organized Violence. San José, Costa Rica, November 27—December 2, 1989

Genefke IK: Reflections concerning torture in the modern world. Copenhagen: Rehabilitation and Research Centre for Torture Victims, 1982

Giller EL: Biological assessment and treatment of posttraumatic stress disorder. Washington, DC, American Psychiatric Press, 1990

Goldfeld AE, Mollica RF, Pesavento BH, et al: The physical and psychological sequelae of torture symptomatology and diagnosis. JAMA 259:2725–2729, 1988

Goldman HH, Goldston SW (eds): Preventing Stress-Related Psychiatric Disorders (DHHS Publ No ADM-85-1366) Washington, DC, U.S. Government Printing Office, 1985

Herman JL: Sequelae of prolonged and repeated trauma: evidence for a complex posttraumatic syndrome (DESNOS), in Posttraumatic Stress Disorder: DSM-IV and Beyond. Edited by Davidson JRT, Foa EB. Washington, DC, American Psychiatric Press, 1993, pp 213–228

Holtan N, Robertson C: Scarcity among plenty: how to treat victims of torture in the USA without government assistance. Torture 2:11, 1992

Jacobsen L, Vesti P: Treatment of torture survivors: the nurse's function. Int Nurs Rev 4:75–80, 1989

Jaranson J: Psychotherapeutic medication, in Mental Health Services for Refugees (DHHS Publ No ADM-91-1824). Edited by Westermeyer J, Williams CL, Nguyen AN. Washington, DC, U.S. Government Printing Office, 1991

Jaranson J: Torture, PTSD and culture. Paper presented at the Scientific Institute on Ethnocultural Aspects of Post-Traumatic Stress and Related Stress Disorders: Issues, Research, and Directions, Honolulu, June 27–July 2, 1993

Jaranson J: Governmental torture: status of the rehabilitation movement. Transcultural Psychiatric Research Review 32:253–286, 1995

Lin KM, Poland RE, Nagasaki G (eds): Psychopharmacology and psychobiology of ethnicity. Washington, DC, American Psychiatric Press, 1993

McCann L, Pearlman LA: Vicarious traumatization: a framework for understanding the psychological effects of working with victims. J Trauma Stress 3:131–148, 1990

Mollica R: The trauma story: the psychiatric care of refugee survivors of violence and torture, in Post-Traumatic Therapy and Victims of Violence. Edited by Ochberg FM. New York, Brunner/Mazel, 1988

Mollica RF, Caspi-Yavin Y: Overview: the assessment and diagnosis of torture events and symptoms, in Torture and Its Consequences: Current Treatment Approaches. Edited by Basoglu M. New York, Cambridge University Press, 1992, pp 253–274

Mollica RF, Wyshak G, Lavelle J, et al: Assessing symptom change in Southeast Asian refugee survivors of mass violence and torture. Am J Psychiatry 147:83–88, 1990

Mollica RF, Caspi-Yavin Y, Bollini P, et al: The Harvard trauma questionnaire: validating a cross-cultural instrument for measuring torture, trauma, and PTSD in Indochinese refugees. J Nerv Ment Dis 180:111–116, 1992

Munoz E: Patient-physician confidentiality on trial in Turkey. JAMA 276:1375–1376, 1996

Murburg MM (ed): Catecholamine Function in Posttraumatic Stress: Emerging Concepts. Washington, DC, American Psychiatric Association, 1994

Nightingale EO: The problem of torture and the response of the health professional, in Health Services for the Treatment of Torture and Trauma Survivors. Edited by Gurschow J, Hannibal K. Washington, DC, American Association for the Advancement of Science, 1990, pp 8–9

Ortmann J, Genefke IK, Jakobsen L, et al: Rehabilitation of torture victims: an interdisciplinary treatment model. American Journal of Social Psychiatry 4:161–167, 1987

Parong AA, Protacio-Marcelino E, Estrado-Claudio S, et al: Rehabilitation of survivors of torture and political violence under a continuing stress situation: the Philippine experience, in Torture and Its Consequences: Current Treatment Approaches. Edited by Basoglu M. New York, Cambridge University Press, 1992, pp 483–510

Physicians for Human Rights: Medical Testimony on Victims of Torture: A Physician's Guide to Political Asylum Cases. Boston, Physicians for Human Rights, 1991

Prip K, Amris K, Marcussen H (eds): Physiotherapy to torture survivors. Torture 4 (suppl 1):3–50, 1994

Randall GR, Lutz EL: Serving survivors of torture. Washington, DC, American Association for the Advancement of Science, 1991

Rasmussen OV: Medical aspects of torture: torture types and their relation to symptoms and lesions in 200 victims, followed by a description of the medical profession in relation to torture. Dan Med Bull 37 (suppl 1):1–88, 1990

Rasmussen OV, Lunde I: Evaluation of investigation of 200 torture victims. Dan Med Bull 27:241–243, 1980

Rasmussen OV, Skylv G: Signs of falanga torture. Torture 3:16–17, 1993

Shapiro F: Eye Movement Desensitization and Reprocessing: Basic Principles, Protocols, and Procedures. New York, Guilford Press, 1995

Simpson MA: Methods of investigating allegations of electric shock torture: lessons from South Africa. Torture 4:27–29, 1994

Skolnick AA: Health care for refugees and survivors of torture is becoming a growth industry, experts sadly say. JAMA 274:288–290, 1995

Skylv G: The physical sequelae of torture, in Torture and Its Consequences: Current Treatment Approaches. Edited by Basoglu M. New York, Cambridge University Press, 1992, pp 38–55

Skylv G: Falange—diagnosis and treatment of late sequelae. Torture 3:11–15, 1993

Solkoff N: The Holocaust: survivors and their children, in Torture and Its Consequences: Current Treatment Approaches. Edited by Basoglu M. New York, Cambridge University Press, 1992, pp 136–148

United Nations: Convention against torture and other cruel, inhuman, or degrading treatment or punishment, in Methods of Combatting Torture. Geneva, United Nations Centre for Human Rights, 1989, p 17

United Nations: Need for international funding of rehabilitation activities for victims of torture worldwide, in Report of the Secretary General, Annex 3, March 21, 1996. Geneva, United Nations Economic and Social Council, 1996 van Willigen LHM: Organization of care and rehabilitation services for victims of torture and other forms of organized violence: a review of current issues, in Torture and Its Consequences: Current Treatment Approaches. Edited by Basoglu M. New York, Cambridge University Press, 1992, pp 277–298

Vesti P, Kastrup K: Psychotherapy for torture survivors, in Torture and Its Consequences: Current Treatment Approaches. Edited by Basoglu M. New York, Cambridge University Press, 1992, pp 348–362

Westermeyer J, Lam L: A review of rehabilitation centers for torture victims. Refugee Mental Health Letter 2:2–5, 1989

Section II

Identifying and Defining Sequelae

CHAPTER 3

Diagnosis of Governmental Torture

Inge Genefke, M.D., D.M.Sc.h.c.
Peter Vesti, M.D.

Physicians have learned much about the documentation of torture based on both physical and psychological sequelae. Examination methods, interview techniques, and data collection have become more sophisticated. Through medical examination, physicians can now detect indications of torture in most of the major organ systems, including the dermatological, cardiopulmonary, gastrointestinal, musculoskeletal, neurological, urological, gynecological, otorhinolaryngological, and ophthalmological systems, as well as in the teeth. Psychological symptoms now fit into the well-defined category of posttraumatic stress disorder (PTSD) as defined by the World Health Organization and the American Psychiatric Association in DSM-IV (American Psychiatric Association 1994). The medical profession's level of sophistication in assessing torture victims has evolved to the extent that the concept of a torture syndrome based on the results of both physical and mental torture has been proposed.

Diagnosing Torture

The recognition of symptomatology related to torture was a phenomenon of the 1970s. At that time, there was no systematic medical literature on torture. Subsequently, we were surprised to encounter a series of findings that were contrary to our expectations.

The first detailed, systematic studies of the methods of torture and its immediate aftereffects were presented by Danish doctors in 1974–1975 (Amnesty International 1977). The work was begun to find forensic medical evidence that torture had occurred. At an early stage, we concluded that the worst sequelae of torture were psychological. That was a first surprise, confirmed by other international studies (Allodi 1980; Forest 1982; Kordon et al. 1988; Rasmussen 1990). Not only is torture unbearable, perverse, and disgusting when it happens, but it stays with survivors and haunts them many years later.

For survivors, deep feelings of guilt and shame often occur after torture. Guilt may be caused by the mere fact of survival. Friends may have died while being tortured, or perhaps information was given that harmed friends. A feeling of guilt may also have social consequences for the family. Guilt may be produced by the so-called impossible choice, in which victims must choose between, for instance, revealing the names of their friends and seeing family members tortured. Regardless of the victim's choice, the result is a disaster for which he or she feels responsible. This is exactly what the torturer wants.

Early studies of survivors of torture at the Rehabilitation and Research Centre for Torture Victims (RCT) revealed the following mental symptoms: anxiety, memory lapses, depression, altered personality, frequent nightmares about prisons and torture, and difficulty in remembering and concentrating (Somnier and Genefke 1986). Fatigue, headache, and sexual disturbances were also common. All these reactions may be considered normal in ordinary people who have been exposed to something as perverse, cruel, and abnormal as torture. These findings have been confirmed by several other studies of victims of torture from all parts of the world (Allodi et al. 1985; Cathcart et al. 1979; Chester 1990; Daly 1980; Domovitch et al. 1984; Fischmann and Ross 1990; Fornazzari and Freire 1990; Forster et al. 1987; Garcia-Peltoniemi 1991; Gonsalves 1990; Hougen et al. 1988; Jaranson 1990; Mollica et al. 1987; Pagaduan-Lopez 1987; Petersen and Jacobsen 1985; Weisæth 1989).

For many years, we have monitored the various forms of torture and their sequelae (Lunde et al. 1992) to understand the frequency and etiology of changes in health after torture. This in turn helps us to identify target groups. We use this information when we set priorities for work in the prevention of torture.

The other main reason for monitoring is to understand better the course of the health consequences of torture. In Table 3–1, we present the psychiatric symptoms most frequently observed by RCT psychotherapists. The location of the symptoms within DSM-IV diagnostic categories is also given. Nine of the most common symptoms are encompassed by the diagnostic criteria for PTSD. It is interesting that symptoms 10 and 11 from our list, that is, *change in personality* and *survivor guilt*, are included under *associated descriptive features* in the entry for PTSD in DSM-IV. They are mentioned among a number of symptoms that are more commonly seen in association with an interpersonal stressor in criterion A.

Consensus Group of the Rehabilitation and Research Centre for Torture Victims

The variability in terminology used in various studies prompted RCT to set up an academic, multidisciplinary consensus group in 1990. Its task has been to define uniform terminology to be used internationally for direct comparison of data (Bøjholm et al. 1992). Our experience at RCT during the last decade, together with the results of epidemiological surveys, has indicated that the most frequent torture-related signs and symptoms can be grouped under a limited number of headings without the complexity of the problem being underestimated.

After carefully examining the available nosological systems, the Consensus Group decided to group the mental symptoms according to DSM-III-R (American Psychiatric Association 1987) (Table 3–2). We divided psychological torture into *weakening procedures* and *personality-destroying procedures*. The purpose of weakening procedures is to teach the victim to be helpless and to create exhaustion. Personality-destroying procedures are characterized by the induction of guilt, fear, and loss of self-esteem (Somnier and Genefke 1986).

Physical torture is administered by physical means, but its main im-

Table 3–1. Twelve major symptoms seen by psychotherapists at RCT and location of symptoms within diagnostic categories of DSM-IV

Symptom	PTSD criterion (DSM-IV)[a]	Description or comment[b]
1. Emotional lability	D2, D4	Irritability or outbursts of anger, hypervigilance
2. Sleep disturbances	B2, D1	Nightmares, difficulty falling asleep or staying asleep
3. Disturbances in ability to concentrate/remember	C3, D3	Psychogenic amnesia, difficulty concentrating
4. Avoidance of thoughts or feelings associated with torture experience	C1	
5. Avoidance of activities or situations that arouse recollections of torture experience	C2	
6. Diminished ability to establish personal relationships	C5, 6	Feelings of detachment or estrangement from others, restricted range of affect
7. Markedly diminished interest in several significant activities	C4	
8. Sense of foreshortened future	C7	
9. Sudden acting or feeling as though torture situation were recurring	B3, 4	Flashbacks occur after exposure to events or environmental stimuli that symbolize or resemble aspect of torture experience
10. Change in personality		
11. Survivor guilt		
12. Anxiety		Anxiety that is specific to torture experience and is neither neurotic nor psychotic

Note. DSM-IV: American Psychiatric Association (1994). RCT = Rehabilitation and Research Centre for Torture Victims; PTSD = posttraumatic stress disorder.
[a]Empty cells indicate that there is no associated DSM-IV diagnostic category.
[b]Empty cells indicate that there is no description/comment.

Table 3–2. Mental symptoms observed in torture victims and grouped according to DSM-III-R

Anxiety symptoms
Behavioral symptoms
Symptoms affecting cognition
Symptoms affecting energy
Symptoms affecting form and amount of thought/speech
Mood/affect disturbance
Occupational and social impairment
Perceptual disturbance (including hallucinations)
Personality trait symptoms
Physical signs and symptoms
Sleep disturbance

pact is of a psychological nature. Physical methods are classified according to the body part afflicted and by the type of trauma mechanism. For the latter, the International Classification of Diseases trauma classification has been adopted. Algorithms for both psychological and physical torture methods have been developed by the RCT Consensus Group (Bøjholm et al. 1992).

Although the mental sequelae of torture can be considered to be largely the same in all torture survivors, physical sequelae depend on the methods used.

We belatedly recognized what was a second surprise: that the ultimate aim of torture is not to obtain information but to break down a person's personality, his or her identity. Toward this goal, torturers destroy their victims' ability to cope with life situations in a normal way. Torture victims have learned their role by heart.

This led us to further analyses and a third surprising discovery: the targets for torturers' destructive work are the so-called strong personalities, people who had displayed the courage and strength to work against repressive regimes. It was much later that we understood that these individuals were a clearly identifiable group. They included union members, fighters for human rights, student leaders, politicians, journalists, and representatives of ethnic minorities. Other people such as common prisoners and demonstrators were also tortured, but the primary targets of governmental torture are the strong personalities.

Finally, our work brought us to a fourth important surprise: we could help the survivors of torture. This still seems a miracle for us. The bullies are not right when they tell the victims of torture that the rest of their lives will be destroyed. The bullies' dirty work can be redressed and remedied (Jacobsen and Vesti 1990).

Does a Torture Syndrome Exist?

We began our work in order to find forensic medical evidence to document that torture had occurred. The question of a possible torture syndrome was raised for the first time by Rasmussen et al. (1977) in 1977 and has been debated during subsequent years. Warmenhoven et al. (1981) concluded in 1981 that the question cannot be answered. Allodi and Cowgill (1982) wrote that the "whole picture constitutes the so-called torture syndrome" (p. 101) and stated that it was similar to PTSD as defined in DSM-III (American Psychiatric Association 1980). However, in a critical review on assessment and treatment of torture victims, Allodi (1991) stated that "more research is needed before valid discrete and specific nosological entities or subcategories of PTSD are created. So far, the 'torture syndrome' remains a cluster of symptoms, sometimes accompanied by more or less specific physical and mental sequelae, subsequent to the unique human-made stressor of torture and included under the general nosological category of PTSD" (Allodi 1991, p. 9).

Yüksel and Kandemir (1991) stated that there are several objections to including torture as a specific form of trauma in medical classification. These objections can be interpreted partly as objections to reduction or medicalization of an essentially sociopolitical problem, as Turner and Gorst-Unsworth (1989) also mentioned. They concluded that although posttraumatic diagnoses and their concordance with PTSD are disputable, the clinical syndromes seen were mostly anxiety disorders and PTSD. However, nearly all of them were chronic, lasting longer than 6 months. At the Center for Victims of Torture in Minnesota, nearly 70% of the clients meet diagnostic criteria for PTSD. Nearly all of the clients exhibit at least one or two symptoms of this disorder (Garcia-Peltoniemi 1990). In 1990, Turner and Gorst-Unsworth (1990) concluded that "the attempts to describe a single 'torture syndrome' . . . are generally unconvincing" (p. 475). Finally, Mollica and Caspi-Yavin (1992), who have considerable experience working with Southeast Asian refugee survivors, concluded that "medical investigations of torture survivors not only failed to demonstrate a unique torture syndrome, but demonstrated symptoms closely associated with the DSM-III-R diagnosis of PTSD" (p. 262). Consequently, investigators have shifted their focus away from demonstrating the presence of a unique syndrome to establishing the prevalence of PTSD in torture survivors, in accordance with the statement by Allodi and Cowgill (1982).

However, the association between PTSD and torture is not a simple linear one. Research by Ramsay et al. (1993) showed that although there is an association between torture and PTSD, different forms of torture produce different PTSD symptoms. More specifically, individuals who had experienced isolation or blindfolding, impact torture, and other physical torture had more PTSD intrusion symptoms, whereas individuals who had been sexually tortured described more avoidance phenomena. This may suggest that PTSD in the cases of tortured individuals is not a uniform syndrome.

Vesti and Kastrup (1995) concluded that a substantial proportion of survivors developed symptomatology similar to that of PTSD but that others did not. This is consistent with our knowledge that there are individual differences in response to severe stress, and we are in the early stages of describing this latter group. Basoglu et al. (1994), for example, documented that perceived severity but not objective severity of torture was associated with PTSD, anxiety, and depression in torture victims. Impact of captivity experience on family was the strongest predictor of PTSD symptoms. Age, personality, previous emotional and physical health, ideological and political commitment, and quality of the posttorture environment can affect the development of PTSD and other symptoms. The presence or absence of social support and the individual's perception of others' helpfulness are important variables for the reduction of the probability of full-blown PTSD (De Silva 1993).

In 1985, Petersen et al. (1985) reexamined 22 Greeks who had been tortured. Eight of them fulfilled the criteria for the chronic organic psychosyndrome. These included symptoms, experienced daily, of at least three of four types: 1) reduced memory or ability to concentrate; 2) disturbances of sleep; 3) emotional lability, anxiety, and depression; and 4) vegetative symptoms of the gastrointestinal or cardiopulmonary systems.

In 1988, RCT and its International Rehabilitation Council for Torture Victims (IRCT) asked centers in other countries for their opinions about a proposed revision of the DSM-III-R diagnosis of PTSD that would include a torture syndrome diagnosis. Responses (not published) were divided for and against this idea. The main arguments against including a torture syndrome diagnosis have been that such a diagnosis 1) would unnecessarily stigmatize the individual and 2) could not reflect all the possible psychiatric and psychological problems that may be seen after torture.

Some centers in developing countries placed an emphasis on the recognition of torture as a medical issue and the need for a formal account of the symptoms that follow severe violations of human rights. These centers pointed out that no compensation is presently given to victims and that there is no understanding in their populations or among their politicians that sequelae of torture exist. Therefore, the diagnosis of posttorture syndrome is important.

Regarding the existence off a torture syndrome, RCT acknowledges that influential researchers on torture have shifted their focus away from a unique torture syndrome and include the psychopathological syndromes following torture as a subtype of the PTSD category. However, the criteria for PTSD are not sufficient for the categorization of the entire picture after torture. The psychological and physical profiles of PTSD and the posttorture state diverge considerably.

Symptoms that are core criteria for the definition of the posttorture state, according to the experience of our team, are described in the DSM-IV definition of PTSD as associated symptoms that are not necessary for a diagnosis of PTSD. These core symptoms are survivors' guilt with low self-esteem, changed personality (the continuity, wholeness, and autonomy of the self is negatively affected), physical sequelae without organic substrate, and many physical complaints without corresponding medical findings. Diffuse pain is a crucial element in the physical and psychological profile of the torture survivor (Juhler and Smidt-Nielsen 1995).

Further research in this field might suggest that when the extreme traumatic stressor is interpersonal (thus a narrower criterion A), the posttorture psychological and physical picture cannot be adequately described by the PTSD entity as it is currently defined. Systematic torture constitutes a more fundamental assault on the individual's self and assumptive world (Janoff-Bulman 1985) than does random violence or other forms of extreme trauma such as natural disasters.

There is therefore a continuing need for specialized research on the hypothesis of a torture syndrome.

Can a Person Who Has Suffered Governmental Torture Be Diagnosed?

We know today that the persons who have experienced governmental torture are strong individuals—people from ethnic minorities, fighters for human rights, politicians, union members, student leaders, and journalists. In other words, there exists a reasonably well-defined group at risk.

We know that those who have been imprisoned in the more than 70 countries in which governmental torture is still practiced (mostly in police stations) suffer from trauma. We know that imprisonment in these countries is often synonymous with torture. We also have knowledge of the methods of torture used and their sequelae. We can, for example, ask the survivor in a medical interview what he or she felt during torture and what coping mechanisms he or she used. We know the symptoms and objective findings that immediately follow torture. For each form of torture, we have detailed knowledge of the development of symptoms. This background can function as a control with regard to the information reported by survivors.

We presently have a wide knowledge of survivors' physical and mental complaints as well as objective findings for these individuals. Thus, survivors of torture make up a population with reasonably well-defined psychological and physical symptoms. The following sections serve to clarify this point.

Psychosomatic Complaints in Torture Victims

Juhler and Smidt-Nielsen (1995) studied 50 survivors of torture to determine whether a typical pattern exists and whether such a pattern could make recognition of the torture survivor more straightforward. These authors noted that there was a discrepancy between the (large) number of physical complaints and the (small) number of objective medical findings, with the exception of musculoskeletal findings, which were evident in each of the 50 individuals examined (Table 3–3).

Table 3–3. Discrepancies between percentage of physical complaints and medical findings in 50 victims of torture

Type of complaint	Complaints (%)	Findings (%)
None	0	4
Neurological	86	22
Cardiopulmonary	74	14
Gastrointestinal	68	24
Urological	34	4
Sexual/genital	54	16
Musculoskeletal	92	92

Although our RCT cohort was seen typically several years after torture, the observed pattern was consistent and striking. The subjects' complaints were psychosomatic, involving perceptions of unresolved mental stress as physical disease in the form of general malaise, diffuse pains, or organ-related complaints. However, these vague and nonspecific complaints and the lack of an organic substrate (which was searched for) are, in reality, the typical hallmarks of the torture survivor.

When a physician is confronted with a person who belongs to one of the aforementioned groups (such as ethnic minorities or fighters for human rights) and who manifests many psychosomatic problems but whose objective findings are primarily related to the musculoskeletal system, the physician should bear in mind that these characteristics are typical of a person who has been exposed to governmental torture.

Physical Abuse:
Specific Symptoms and Objective Findings

Beatings

Falanga is the beating of the soles of the feet with cables, iron, sticks, or other instruments of wood or metal. Victims are usually restrained with the feet raised. There are many different ways to administer falanga.

The immediate symptoms after falanga are swelling of the feet, ankles, and lower legs. Subsequently, the skin may slough. Late symptoms of falanga include pain in the legs and feet, mainly deep in the tibial region and near the joints. This pain is described as jabbing, cutting, or burning. It may be constant, but it is usually intermittent. There is often a direct relationship between the pain and the act of walking or running. The rate of walking is slow and the distance traveled is limited. Now and then, victims must stop and sit down before continuing. They cannot sit with crossed legs or squat. The pain is worse in cold, damp, and windy weather. There may be sensations of tiredness and heaviness in the thighs and legs and sensations of looseness in the knees and ankles, as if the joints were falling apart. The victims often note that their gait has changed. The feet cannot move freely; they cannot be flexed properly. There is often lower back pain during standing or walking, but the typical radiating pains of nerve irritation are absent. There is little or limited swelling of the ankles and feet.

On inspection, the pads of the heels and the medial and lateral balls of the forefeet may appear smashed. These are signs of severe edema immediately after the torture, in which the vertical connective tissue trabeculae from the skin to the bones between the fat pockets are torn. This causes the balls of the feet to lose their spring and thus their function as shock absorbers. As a result, the pressure produced when the feet hit the ground during walking is transmitted unimpeded through the long bones and the joints to the spine, causing lower back pain during walking. Injury to the balls of the forefeet should be considered indicative of falanga. Smashed heel pads can be diagnosed in several ways. The condition is similar to that seen in long-distance runners in whom only the pads of the heels are injured. The skin of the soles often shows hard, rough scars. These lead to the adoption of a pathological gait to give pain relief. The symptoms may resemble reflex sympathetic dystrophy (RSD). There is often increased sweating and altered temperature perception, but other signs of RSD, such as reduced hair growth and pointed toes, are missing.

On palpation, the entire length of the plantar aponeurosis is tender and feels rough, as in the case of tendinitis caused by overexercise. Passive extension of the big toe will reveal whether the aponeurosis has been torn. If it is intact, one should feel the start of tension in the aponeurosis on palpation when the toe is bent backward 20 degrees. The maximum normal extension is 70 degrees. Higher values suggest injury of the attachment of the aponeurosis.

Passive movement of the small joints of the feet usually shows joint stiffness and decreased movement in many of them. During falanga, as in a hard landing on the heels, the talus is forced up against the tibia. This trauma and the accompanying edema result in overstretching of the stabilizing ligaments around the ankle, compromising the normal shock-absorbent and stabilizing function of the connection between tibia and fibula (Skylv 1992).

Clinical examination reveals tenderness of both the superior and inferior tibiofibular joints. There is indirect tenderness of these joints when pressure from below is placed on the tuber calcanei (Amris et al. 1995).

Lök et al. (1991) published findings relating to falanga. Five cases of falanga have been studied using bone scintigraphy, which may be a sensitive indicator of trauma. This technique may reveal small fractures missed by conventional radiography. Scintigraphy repeated more than 5 months later may produce similar positive results. Given that our patients did not have fractures corresponding to the active scintigraphic site, the scans may have been revealing periosteal damage caused by the beatings (Lök 1993; Lök et al. 1991).

In summary, we know the methods of falanga, the symptoms (immediate and late), the objective findings (immediate and late), the results of bone scintigraphy of feet affected by falanga, and the changes produced by falanga. Therefore, we can diagnose falanga with great certainty.

Other forms of beatings include mechanical acceleration-deceleration effects on the vertebral column that cause whiplash syndrome. Such an injury is an example of musculoskeletal injuries' causing not only widespread physical symptoms but also psychological disabilities (Amris 1995).

Suspension

Examples of objective findings after other forms of torture include shoulder joint pain, often radiating down into the arms, caused by suspension by the arms. Also in victims of this type of suspension, the joints to the thorax are strained and cause localized precordial pain, which is often misinterpreted as heart pain. A special form of suspension, the Palestinian hanging, may cause lesions of the brachial plexus, leading to neurogenic pain (Jacobsen and Smidt-Nielsen 1996; A. B. Thomsen et al. 1981).

Electrical Torture

The sequelae and scientific proof of electrical torture have been described thoroughly (Danielsen 1992; Danielsen and Aalund 1991; Danielsen et al. 1991; Karlsmark et al. 1984; H. K. Thomsen et al. 1981). One specific sequela of electrical torture is alopecia (Piniou-Kalli and Tsikolis 1992).

Altered Sleep Patterns

A main complaint of torture survivors is sleep disturbance, including nightmares, insomnia, and daytime fatigue. Seven subjects who had been exposed to torture were examined by polysomnography (Åstrøm et al. 1989). All had abnormal sleep patterns compared with normal controls matched for age and sex. We found reduced rapid-eye-movement (REM) sleep duration, absent stage 4 sleep, reduction in total sleep, and low sleep efficiency. None of these torture victims had depression, and none had the short REM sleep latency that is a characteristic finding in endogenous depression.

Conclusion

A clear portrait of the survivors of governmental torture has emerged. In the at-risk groups, we find individuals who feel themselves changed after being in police stations or prisons. They feel different, no longer recognize themselves, and consider themselves changed in activity and interest. They react to very specific provocative factors with anxiety attacks.

After almost 20 years of medical work against torture, we note that those exposed to governmental torture represent a predictable risk group experiencing reasonably well-defined physical and psychological sequelae. Future research will refine the significant divergences between PTSD and the posttorture syndrome. Today we are able to state with confidence whether a person is a survivor of governmental torture.

References

Allodi F: The psychiatric effects in children and families of victims of political persecution and torture. Dan Med Bull 27:229–232, 1980

Allodi F: Assessment and treatment of torture victims: a critical review. J Nerv Ment Dis 179:4–11, 1991

Allodi F, Cowgill G: Ethical and psychiatric aspects of torture: a Canadian study. Can J Psychiatry 27:98–102, 1982

Allodi F, Randall GR, Lutz EL, et al: Physical and psychiatric effects of torture: two medical studies, in The Breaking of Bodies and Minds: Torture, Psychiatric Abuse and the Health Professions. Edited by Stover E, Nightingale EO. New York, WH Freeman, 1985, pp 58–78

American Psychiatric Association: Diagnostic and Statistical Manual of Mental Disorders, 3rd Edition. Washington, DC, American Psychiatric Association, 1980

American Psychiatric Association: Diagnostic and Statistical Manual of Mental Disorders, 3rd Edition, Revised. Washington, DC, American Psychiatric Association, 1987

American Psychiatric Association: Diagnostic and Statistical Manual of Mental Disorders, 4th Edition. Washington, DC, American Psychiatric Association, 1994

Amnesty International. Evidence of Torture: Studies by the Amnesty International Danish Medical Group. London, Amnesty International Publications, 1977

Amris K: The whiplash syndrome, in Physiotherapy for Torture Survivors: A Basic Introduction. Edited by Prip K, Tived L, Holten N. Copenhagen, International Rehabilitation Council for Torture Victims, 1995

Amris K, Prip K, Tived L: Diagnostic Considerations and Treatment After Falanga Torture. Copenhagen, RCT/IRCT, 1995

Åstrøm C, Lunde I, Ortmann J, et al: Sleep disturbances in torture survivors. Acta Neurol Scand 79:150–154, 1989

Basoglu M, Paker M, Özmen E, et al: Factors related to long-term traumatic stress responses in survivors of torture in Turkey. JAMA 272:357–363, 1994

Bøjholm S, Foldspang A, Juhler M, et al: Monitoring the Health and Rehabilitation of Torture Survivors: A Management Information System for a Rehabilitation and Research Unit for Torture Victims. Copenhagen, Rehabilitation and Research Centre for Torture Victims, 1992

Cathcart IM, Berger P, Knazan B: Medical examination of torture victims applying for refugee status. Can Med Assoc J 121:179–184, 1979

Chester B: Because mercy has a human heart: centers for victims of torture, in Psychology and Torture. Edited by Suedfeld P. New York, Hemisphere, 1990, pp 165–184

Daly RJ: Compensation and rehabilitation of victims of torture: an example of preventative psychiatry. Dan Med Bull 27:245–248, 1980

Danielsen L: Scientific proof of electric torture. Interpol International Criminal Police Review 436:15–16, 1992

Danielsen L, Aalund O: How electrical torture can be scientifically proved. Torture 3:16–17, 1991

Danielsen L, Karlsmark T, Thomsen HK, et al: Diagnosis of electrical skin injuries: a review and a description of a case. Am J Forensic Med Pathol 12:222–226, 1991

De Silva P: Post-traumatic stress disorder: cross-cultural aspects. International Review of Psychiatry 5:217–229, 1993

Domovitch E, Berger PB, Wawer MJ, et al: Human torture: description and sequelae of 104 cases. Can Fam Physician 30:827–830, 1984

Fischmann Y, Ross J: Group treatment of exiled survivors of torture. Am J Orthopsychiatry 60:135–141, 1990

Forest E: Analisis de la democracia a traves de la tortura, in Tortura y Sociedad. Edited by Cueva J, Morales JL, Grupo de Medicos contra la Tortura, et al. Madrid, Editorial Revolucíon, pp 77–100, 1982

Fornazzari X, Freire M: Women as victims of torture. Acta Psychiatr Scand 82:257–260, 1990

Forster D, Davis D, Sandler D: Detention and Torture in South Africa: Psychological, Legal and Historical Studies. Cape Town, South Africa, David Phillip, 1987

Garcia-Peltoniemi RE: Forgetting and remembering: balancing the needs of society and the individual. Paper presented at the 6th annual meeting of the International Society for Traumatic Stress Studies, New Orleans, LA, October 28–31, 1990

Garcia-Peltoniemi RE: Clinical manifestations of psychopathology, in Refugee Mental Health Program: Mental Health Services for Refugees (DHHS Publ No ADM-91-1824). Rockville, MD, National Institute of Mental Health, 1991, pp 42–55

Gonsalves CJ: The psychological effects of political repression on Chilean exiles in the US. Am J Orthopsychiatry 60:143–153, 1990

Hougen HP, Kelstrup J, Peterson HD, et al: Sequelae to torture: a controlled study of torture victims living in exile. Forensic Sci Int 36:153–160, 1988

Jacobsen L, Smidt-Nielsen K: Torturoverlever—traume og rehabilitering. Copenhagen, RCT, 1996

Jacobsen L, Vesti P: Torture Survivors: A New Group of Patients. Copenhagen, Danish Nurses' Organization, 1990

Janoff-Bulman R: The aftermath of victimization: rebuilding shattered assumptions, in Trauma and Its Wake: The Study and Treatment of Post-Traumatic Stress Disorders. Edited by Figley CR. New York, Brunner/Mazel, 1985

Jaranson JM: Mental health treatment of refugees and immigrants, in Mental Health of Immigrants and Refugees: Proceedings of a Conference Sponsored by Hogg Foundation for Mental Health and World Foundation for Mental Health. Edited by Holtzman WH, Bornemann TH. Austin, TX, Hogg Foundation for Mental Health, 1990, pp 207–215

Juhler M, Smidt-Nielsen K: Identification of torture survivors: a comparative study of medical complaints and findings in torture survivors. Abstracts of papers presented at the VIIth International Symposium in Caring for Survivors of Torture: Challenges for the Medical and Health Professions, Cape Town, South Africa, November 15–17, 1995

Karlsmark T, Thomsen HK, Danielsen L, et al: Tracing the use of electrical torture. Am J Forensic Med Pathol 5:333–337, 1984

Kordon DR, Edelman LI, Lagos DM, et al: Psychological effects of political repression. Buenos Aires, Argentina, Sudamerica/Planeta, 1988

Lök V: Determination of a permanent evidence of torture by scintigraphy, in European Parliament: Summary Record of Presentations Made at the Public Hearing on the Fight Against Torture and the Role of Rehabilitation Centres. Brussels, Committee on Foreign Affairs and Security, Subcommittee on Human Rights, December 20–21, 1993

Lök V, Tunca M, Kumanlioglu K, et al: Bone scintigraphy as clue to previous torture. Lancet 337:846–847, 1991

Lunde I, Foldspang A, Hansen AH, et al: Monitoring the health of torture victims: a pilot study, in Health Situation of Refugees and Victims of Organized Violence. Edited by van Willigen L. Rijswijk, The Netherlands: Ministry of Welfare, Health and Cultural Affairs, 1992, pp 117–135

Mollica RF, Caspi-Yavin Y: Overview: the assessment and diagnosis of torture events and symptoms, in Torture and Its Consequences: Current Treatment Approaches. Edited by Basoglu M. New York, Cambridge University Press, 1992, pp 253–274

Mollica RF, Wyshak G, Lavelle J: The psychosocial impact of war trauma and torture on Southeast Asian refugees. Am J Psychiatry 144:1567–1572, 1987

Pagaduan-Lopez JC: Torture Survivors: What Can We Do for Them? Manila, The Philippines, Medical Action Group, 1987

Petersen HD, Jacobsen P: Psychological and physical symptoms after torture: A prospective controlled study. Forensic Sci Int 29:179–189, 1985

Petersen HD, Abildgaard U, Daugaard G, et al: Psychological and long-term effects of torture: a follow-up examination of 22 Greek persons exposed to torture, 1967–1974. Scand J Soc Med 13:89–93, 1985

Piniou-Kalli M, Tsikolis P: Alopecia after electroshocks: traumatic or psychogenic? Paper presented at the Vth International Symposium on Torture and the Medical Profession, Istanbul, Turkey, October 22–24, 1992

Ramsay R, Gorst-Unsworth C, Turner S: Psychiatric morbidity in survivors of organised state violence including torture. A retrospective series. Br J Psychiatry 162:55–59, 1993

Rasmussen OV: Medical aspects of torture: torture types and their relation to symptoms and lesions in 200 victims, followed by a description of the medical profession in relation to torture. Dan Med Bull 37 (suppl 1):1–88, 1990

Rasmussen OV, Dam AM, Nielsen IL: Torture: a study of Chilean and Greek victims, in Evidence of Torture: Studies by the Amnesty International Danish Medical Group. London, Amnesty International Publications, 1977, pp 9–19

Skylv G: The physical sequelae of torture. In Torture and Its Consequences: Current Treatment Approaches. Edited by Basoglu M. New York, Cambridge University Press, 1992, pp 38–55

Somnier FE, Genefke IK: Psychotherapy for victims of torture. Br J Psychiatry 149:323–329, 1986

Thomsen AB, Eriksen J, Smidt-Nielsen K: Neurogene smerter efter palæstinensisk hængning. Ugeskr Læger 159(4):129–130, 1997

Thomsen HK, Danielsen L, Nielsen O, et al: Early epidermal changes in heat and electrically injured pig skin, I: a light microscopic study. Forensic Sci Int 17:133–143, 1981

Turner S, Gorst-Unsworth C: Reactions to torture: psychological, political and social issues. Paper presented at the International Conference of Centres, Institutions and Individuals Concerned With the Care of Victims of Organized Violence, San Jose, Costa Rica, November 27–December 2, 1989

Turner S, Gorst-Unsworth C: Psychological sequelae of torture: a descriptive model. Br J Psychiatry 157:475–480, 1990

Vesti P, Kastrup M: Refugee status, torture, and adjustment, in Traumatic Stress: From Theory to Practice. Edited by Freedy JR. London, Plenum Press, 1995, pp 213–235

Warmenhoven C, van Slooten H, Lachinsky N, et al: Medische gevolgen van martelingen: enn onderzoek bij vluchtelingen in Nederland. Ned Tijdschr Geneeskd 125:104–108, 1981

Weisæth L: Torture of a Norwegian ship's crew: the torture, stress reactions and psychiatric after-effects. Acta Psychiatr Scand 80:63–72, 1989

Yüksel S, Kandemir E: Does only PTSD develop after being exposed to torture? Paper presented at conference entitled Conceptualizing Anxiety in Torture Survivors, Copenhagen, September 20–21, 1991

CHAPTER 4

Three Categories of Victimization Among Refugees in a Psychiatric Clinic

Joe Westermeyer, M.D., Ph.D.
Mark Williams, M.D.

In this chapter, we discuss refugees who were psychiatric patients at a university department of psychiatry, and we emphasize the types and correlates of victimization. In today's shrinking world, clinicians in virtually any medical setting can encounter victims among their patients. Such victims of traumatic experiences include torture survivors, refugees, combat veterans, concentration camp survivors, rape victims, and survivors of man-made and natural disasters. Knowledge of the presenting signs and symptoms, likely complications or sequelae, and the means of assessment needed for aiding such persons has become a necessity.

The magnitude of victimization in the world today is often not appreciated. Considering refugees alone, approximately 18 million displaced persons now exist. According to Amnesty International (1994), torture still occurs in 98 countries at present. More than 100 million people living today have been refugees at some time in their lives, and many are survivors of torture. Approximately 18% of the American population today is foreign born; many of these persons have come to the United States as refugees, from World War II to the present (Bacon 1998).

Review of Literature on Trauma

The literature indicates psychiatric similarities among victims regardless of the source of trauma. The diagnostic term *posttraumatic stress disorder* (PTSD) became an official diagnosis in 1980 with the publication of DSM-III (American Psychiatric Association 1980). This term replaced earlier descriptive terms such as *combat fatigue* and *battle stress*.

In the Epidemiologic Catchment Area study (Helzer et al. 1987), PTSD was found to have 6-month prevalence rates of 1% in the native-born population, compared with 3.5% in civilians exposed to physical attack or in Vietnam veterans who were not wounded and 20% in veterans wounded in battle. Even higher rates have been found in clinical populations such as prisoners of war (POWs). For example, Speed et al. (1989) found that 50% of 62 former World War II POWs met criteria for PTSD in the first year after repatriation. Kluznik et al. (1986) studied 188 former POWs and found that 67% had PTSD. Similarly, the frequency of PTSD is greater among clinical populations of refugees than in the general population. For example, Mollica et al. (1987) studied 52 patients in a clinic for Indochinese refugees and found that 50% met criteria for PTSD. Similar rates were found among immigrants from Central America and Mexico in a study by Cervantes et al. (1989).

ᐰ Information about the role of demographics in the reaction to trauma is limited. Some studies have suggested that culture or race may have an effect on either the victimization process itself or the ability or opportunity to recover. For example, Kinzie et al. (1990) found a higher rate of PTSD among mountaineer Mien refugees from the hills of Laos than among lowland Vietnamese refugees (93% versus 54%). Mollica et al. (1987) noted that refugee Cambodian women without husbands demonstrated more serious psychiatric and social impairments than did all other Indochinese patient groups. Other studies have associated gender with the type of torture experienced, with sexual abuse noted to be more frequent among female victims of torture (Allodi and Stiasny 1990). Widowhood has been correlated with higher numbers of symptoms of depression and anxiety among Asian refugees (Kroll et al. 1989). Advanced age, female gender, and the diagnosis of depression were correlated with a higher prevalence of PTSD in one refugee group (Kinzie et al. 1990).

Several other psychiatric sequelae of trauma have accompanied PTSD. However, reports from the literature differ with regard to the distribution of associated psychiatric symptoms and disorders. For example, Helzer et al. (1987) found that those with PTSD were twice as likely to have obsessive-compulsive disorder, dysthymia, or bipolar disorder. No increased association was found with schizophrenia, anorexia nervosa, organic mental disorder, or, among men, phobias and panic. In a study of 426 former POWs, Eberly and Engdahl (1991) noted increases in lifetime prevalence rates of major depressive disorder and PTSD, but the rates of schizophrenia, bipolar disorder, and alcoholism were not elevated. In the study by Kroll et al. (1989) of 404 Southeast Asian refugees at a community clinic, three-quarters met DSM-III criteria for major depressive disorder and 14% had PTSD. Somatization was somewhat less frequent among lowland Cambodian and Lao patients than among the mountaineer Hmong. This difference was thought to be related to differing worldviews associated with Buddhism versus animism. Mellman et al. (1992) found that among 60 veteran outpatients who had been exposed to severe combat stress, PTSD was the most prevalent lifetime disorder, followed by major depressive disorder, panic disorder, generalized anxiety disorder, and phobic disorder. An earlier onset of generalized anxiety disorder was thought to represent a primary response to trauma, to be followed later by full-blown PTSD.

Several attempts have been made to correlate Axis II with victimization to identify possible vulnerability versus protective qualities associated with personality factors. In the epidemiological study of native-born Americans (Helzer et al. 1987), behavioral problems before age 15 predicted adult exposure to physical attack, as well as development of PTSD in those so exposed. On the other hand, Solkoff et al. (1986) found no relationship between earlier preservice experiences and subsequent development of PTSD among 50 Vietnam combat veterans diagnosed with PTSD as compared with combat veterans without that diagnosis. Ford and Spauldy (1973), in a study of 82 surviving crew members of the U.S.S. *Pueblo,* noted that those with dependent or obsessive-compulsive characteristics tolerated the POW stresses poorly, compared with crew members with healthy personalities or schizoid personalities. The researchers found no differences in Minnesota Multiphasic Personality Inventory (MMPI) scores between the group that did well and the group that did not.

Axis III medical conditions associated with victimization have varied with the type of victimization. Rasmussen and Lunde (1980) have thoroughly reviewed the medical sequelae of torture. Investigators of the sequelae of torture have examined sleep disorders (Peters et al. 1990), central nervous system changes (Jensen et al. 1982), sexual dysfunction (Lunde et al. 1981), head injury (Goldfeld et al. 1988), and weight loss (Eberly and Engdahl 1991). Torture can have prolonged and extensive effects on health.

Researchers have suggested that the following variables can be used to gauge the neuropsychiatric effects of victimization: 1) the number of days spent in an institution in which torture is used, 2) the percentage of body weight lost during the period of torture, and 3) the number of incidents of unconsciousness during the torture period. The severity of stress among POWs has been associated with the persistence of symptoms (Speed et al. 1989). Among Jewish Holocaust survivors, length of imprisonment has been associated with sleep disturbances and the frequency of nightmares (Rosen et al. 1991). Among Indochinese refugees, extent of victimization has been related to depressive, somatic, and anxiety symptoms (Kroll et al. 1989). Kroll and co-workers (1989) found that those with focused traumatic experiences had worse symptoms than those who had not been captured, assaulted, sent to reeducation camps, or traumatized during their escape. A thorough history of victimization as well as a thorough examination of the neurological-neuroendocrine-neuropsychiatric systems is necessary to assess the sequelae of trauma.

In previous decades, it had been assumed that battle fatigue or other posttraumatic conditions resolved rapidly and spontaneously, much like an adjustment disorder. However, numerous studies indicate that posttraumatic stress symptoms can persist for years or even decades after the traumatic event (Speed et al. 1989; Sutker et al. 1991). Vietnam veterans and refugees alike have shown persistent difficulties in finding steady employment and in maintaining marriages and families as they try to cope with the sequelae of their traumas.

Concern that health professionals are not likely to be aware of victimization because of naïveté or discomfort on their part or discomfort on the part of the victim has produced attempts at professional education and at developing clinical guidelines for evaluation (Westermeyer 1989a, 1989b; Westermeyer and Wahmenholm 1989). The evaluation and treatment of victims can be difficult. Health care providers have often been unprepared for or unresponsive to the needs of victims. At the same time, victims generally do not seek help in a direct manner. Both victim and provider may withdraw from the trauma in fear, horror, disgust, and anger. The evaluation process involves 1) sensitive, properly timed questioning of patients at risk regarding victimization, because of previous victimization; and 2) the use of the multiaxial DSM-IV (American Psychiatric Association 1994) system in making a complete psychiatric diagnosis. Ethical issues are a major part of these clinical endeavors (Allodi and Cowgill 1982).

Background for Current Study

All of the 286 subjects in our study were patients voluntarily seeking care in the International Clinic at the University of Minnesota in Minneapolis. More than 90% of patients were initially evaluated as outpatients. Most patients came from Minnesota and parts of Wisconsin and Iowa. Only refugees were included in this study (nonrefugee immigrants, foreign students, and others were excluded). These study patients were referred largely by other refugees and by various associations, agencies, and clinics that provided services to refugees. We routinely inquired about potential sources of violence in the country of origin, during flight out of the refugee's country, in the country of temporary refuge, and in the United States. Type of victimization concentrated on in this study was restricted to victimization occurring in the country of origin and during refugee flight. A few cases of victimization did occur in the first country of refuge and in the United States, but the numbers were too small to analyze and the data were not included in the study.

Demographic data were obtained in almost all cases by a staff person of the same ethnicity as the patient. Exceptions included the seven patients belonging to non-Indochinese ethnicities. Clinical data came from a clinical team composed of a psychiatrist and an interpreter who interviewed the patient in the patient's native language. The team used several scheduled interview formats (i.e., Hopkins Symptom Checklist—90

[SCL-90-R] [Derogatis 1983], Hamilton Rating Scale for Depression [HRSD] [Hamilton 1960], Hamilton Anxiety Scale [HAS] [Hamilton 1959], Brief Psychiatric Rating Scale [BPRS] [Overall and Gorham 1962], and Global Assessment Scale [GAS] [Spitzer et al. 1973]), and unscheduled interviewing and medical evaluation were performed as well. The process of evaluation did not depend solely on the first interview session but ordinarily proceeded over several weeks, involving several hours or more of patient interviewing and collateral sources of information.

It had been our clinical impression that patients who had been deliberately harmed while incarcerated suffered greater psychological effects than those who had been harmed in an impersonal manner (e.g., during combat, in attacks on villages, in attacks on fleeing persons). Thus we categorized 286 sequential refugee patients based on whether they had experienced deliberate face-to-face harm or threat of harm while incarcerated, impersonal harm or threat of harm while in combat or fleeing, or no harm or threat of harm.

Category One:
Deliberate Violence During Incarceration

Sixteen of 286 patients (5.6%) experienced deliberate face-to-face victimization.

Definition

Face-to-face harm or the threat of harm had been experienced by patients in this category, which consisted of captives, internees, prisoners, or others unable to flee or to protect themselves. *Harm* included beatings, systematized torture, rape, painful binding, starving, social isolation, and incarceration in unhygienic settings. *Threats* included mock executions, even after actual executions of others, and threats on the life of the victim or significant others.

Discussion of Patients

Case Example 1

A Hmong family was captured by Communist Lao soldiers as the family was preparing to cross the Mekong River. Soldiers began systematically beating the family with the butts of their rifles. The father and two children died at the site. The mother and one son were brought by Lao villagers to a local hospital. Both mother and son remained unconscious for several days but survived. The son, previously the brightest offspring, was notably duller after the injury. At the time of our evaluation, the 11-year-old son had been unable to learn English and had other learning disorder symptoms. A skull X ray revealed an old skull fracture, and language-fair intelligence testing demonstrated an IQ consistent with that of a person with a chronological age of 6 years. This boy improved with academic tutoring and parental counseling, both directed at setting expectations consistent with his remaining intellectual capacity.

Case Example 2

A 42-year-old South Vietnamese woman with relatives in the government and the military was imprisoned for several weeks by the Communist government in 1975. During this time she was beaten, starved, and systematically shocked with electricity near her breasts while being questioned by military and civilian intelligence officers of the new regime. Her nephew was killed in front of her by a bullet to the head. Immediately afterward, the same revolver was placed to the patient's head, the hammer was pulled back, and the trigger was pulled, but the chamber was empty. She was also starved and kept isolated in a small, dark cell under unhygienic conditions. Her husband died during the same incarceration.

Following her release, she began to develop depressive and post-traumatic stress symptoms. Several years later, when she joined surviving relatives in the United States, she had major depression with mood-congruent psychotic features and PTSD. Antidepressant medications provided only partial relief, despite adequate trials with several regimens over several months. She eventually recovered after a course of electroconvulsive therapy (ECT). Because of the patient's experience of electrical torture, special education was needed and extra time was spent on other therapies before she and her family could accept ECT. (The 57-year-old Cambodian woman described in Case Example 4, who had not been tortured with electricity, was instrumental—along with her family—in educating several patients and their families about ECT.)

Case Example 3

A 48-year-old South Vietnamese official was incarcerated at the time of the regime change in 1975. He remained incarcerated for the next 11 years. During this time he was exposed to numerous assaults and threats. He endured systematic torture with beatings and the use of electricity during questioning; beatings to the head, resulting in periods of unconsciousness ranging from minutes to hours, as well as two open scalp wounds, each several centimeters in length; starving; and a disease endemic among the prisoners at the camp and marked by diarrhea, confusion, and dermatitis of the face (most of the prisoners in the camp died after contracting the disease, probably pellagra, which is associated with niacin deficiency).

After his release, he joined his family in the United States, but his familial and vocational adjustments went poorly, despite the fact that he had previously received a college education and was fluent in English. On evaluation, he was found to be disoriented for time, with impaired immediate and recent memory, problems with simple subtraction, and an inability to replicate two pentagons intersecting in a trapezoid. Magnetic resonance imaging (MRI) revealed several areas of cortical loss. In addition, he had symptoms of depression and posttraumatic stress. He subsequently did well with lowered family and social agency expectations, the acquisition of Social Security disability benefits, supportive psychotherapy, a course of antidepressant medications, and rehabilitation in a day program.

Case Example 4

A 57-year-old Cambodian woman, brought in to the clinic by her children, had been mentally ill and totally disabled since the Pol Pot era a decade earlier. She had been present when her husband died of starvation, and her sister had been murdered in the same commune. Several other relatives had never been heard from again. However, her two children survived and brought her to the United States.

On interview, she had racing thoughts, auditory hallucinations, and delusions of boundless powers, and she smiled constantly. History obtained from the family revealed marked insomnia, constant but purposeless and sometimes dangerous activities (e.g., "cooking" clothes on the stove, mixing rice with soap powder to eat), and denial regarding the family's past losses and degradations. Trial with several antimanic medications over a 1-year period produced only mild symptomatic improvement. A course of six ECT treatments entirely relieved her manic condition. During the subsequent 2 years of monitoring, she did well on a regimen of psychotherapy for missed bereavement and posttraumatic stress disorder.

These four patients had been previously evaluated and treated by others, but generally a trauma history had not been elicited and a complete bio-psychosocial assessment had not been conducted. Earlier clinical histories in these four cases were as follows:

- The 11-year-old boy, injured at age 8, had been evaluated by a school psychologist and by a pediatrician, both of whom had experience with Indochinese refugee children. They had assessed the child as having a family problem due to a mother who spoke only Hmong at home and who was unable to control her child. They had failed to obtain historical information regarding the head injury or to demonstrate the extent of the child's brain injury.
- The 42-year-old woman had been treated for several months in a sociolegal program for victims of torture. Although the staff had elicited the torture history, they had not conducted a diagnostic evaluation. Treated with group therapy aimed at reliving and integrating the torture experience, this woman deteriorated during her group treatment. Alarmed, the family had sought other help through their refugee association.
- The 48-year-old man had been under the aegis of a religious refugee-relocation agency for several months before his evaluation. Despite the agency's failure to rehabilitate the man, no psychiatric or medical consultation was sought. Eventually, the family, on the verge of turning him out of the household, was persuaded by a Vietnamese refugee association to seek psychiatric assistance.
- The 57-year-old Cambodian woman was referred by her relocation agency when the family complained to the agency about her behavior (her need for constant surveillance was preventing members from working and attending school). Other than being given herbal nostrums and shamanistic healing, she had not been previously assessed or treated for her condition.

Demographics

Victims of deliberate physical abuse and threat tended to be older than patients in the other two groups, with a mean age of 44.2 years (SD 14.7

years). Among lowland Southeast Asians (i.e., Lao, Vietnamese, and Cambodians), 12% (13 of 113) were in this group, whereas only 2% (3 of 167) of Hmong were in this group.

None of the refugees from areas of the world besides Southeast Asia were in this group. The number of Cambodians was too small for statistical measures to be applied, but it appeared that they were more likely to be in this group. Three of 8 Cambodian patients were in this category, compared with 13 of 286 for the remaining patients. There was a slight predominance of male patients (10 men and 6 women). Fourteen of the 16 had been married, although 5 were now widowed and 3 were separated or divorced.

Clinical Characteristics

Clinical evaluation revealed a high rate of mood disorder (12 of 16) and psychoactive substance use disorder (4 of 16). The rate of PTSD at the time of the initial evaluation was 25%, although a few additional patients subsequently developed PTSD symptoms once their psychosis was alleviated. Associated medical conditions were frequent, occurring in 10 of these 16 patients. These latter conditions were often associated directly with the patients' mistreatment (e.g., brain damage, poorly mended fractures, peripheral nerve damage), although some illnesses may or may not have been related to maltreatment during confinement (e.g., hypertension).

At the time of the initial evaluation of the patients in this group, the Axis V (DSM-III-R [American Psychiatric Association 1987]) "highest level of coping in the last year" was 4.3 (SD 1.0), which lies between fair (4.0) and poor (5.0). After treatment, coping range was judged to be from "fair" to "very good" (i.e., 2 to 4, on a scale of 1 to 6).

Treatment

Treatment tended to be lengthy in these cases, generally ranging from several months to a few years. Typically, a wide spectrum of treatment modalities was necessary. These modalities included the following:

- Biological treatments: antidepressant medications, antimanic medications, ECT, antianxiety medications (benzodiazepines and other addicting sedatives were avoided because of the risk of iatrogenic psychoactive substance use disorder), withdrawal treatment for substance dependence, anticonvulsants, antihypertensives

- Psychotherapies: supportive therapy; abreactive-integrative therapy; individual therapy; family therapy; behavioral modification therapy, including desensitization; paradoxical therapy; psychodynamic therapy
- Other: day program; inpatient treatment; special education program; consultation with physicians in medicine, neurology, clinical psychology, and pediatrics and with clinical psychologists

One patient in this group failed to show any improvement. This 48-year-old Cambodian woman had previously been treated at another facility with individual and group psychotherapy, during which her condition had progressively deteriorated. She had a major depression with mood-congruent psychotic features. Her husband, two of her four children, and most of her relatives had died during the Pol Pot regime. Several friends and family members had been murdered in her presence, and she had been raped on several occasions. She had been beaten about the head and had been malnourished. She did not comply with evaluation or with several antidepressant medication regimens, and she refused hospitalization despite failed outpatient treatment.

A major consideration in the care of these patients was the timing of various treatment interventions, because all required more than one treatment modality. For example, abreactive-integrative psychotherapy that focused on the victimization was not helpful for a suicidal, melancholic, or psychotic patient. Antidepressant medication therapy was delayed in one case until cardiac assessment had been completed. In many instances, medication prescribed by other services needed to be changed so that medications with known depressive or addictive effects could be avoided. Several of these patients required inpatient care. These complex cases involved psychiatric, neuropsychiatric, biomedical, family, and cultural factors, which interacted in complex ways to produce severe discomfort and disability.

Category Two: Impersonal Violence

Sixty-three of the 286 patients (22.0%) were exposed to impersonal violence during combat, during attacks on their home community, or during refugee flight.

Definition

In this group were individuals who underwent harm or the threat of harm arising as a result of an impersonal assault in which the victims were able to fight back or to escape. Examples included military combat and attacks on communities or on fleeing refugees. Instruments of assault included gunshot, artillery, aerial bombing, and aerial toxins. Some victims were wounded or otherwise injured, some lost friends or relatives, and others were exposed to the threat of injury or death but were not harmed physically.

Discussion of Patients

Case Example 1

A 13-year-old Vietnamese boy was evaluated for failure to learn English. As in the first case example in the group of patients who experienced deliberate violence during incarceration, a pediatrician and a school psychologist had evaluated the patient. They had referred him to our psychiatric clinic because they thought that there might be a psychological block or the patient might be oppositional.

When we were obtaining the patient's history, the parents recalled that the patient had a forehead injury from a mortar attack on their town several years earlier. The boy had been hospitalized for a few weeks, but the family had not received further information regarding the nature of the injury. Following the injury, the boy was noted to do less well in school, to respond less well to correction, to have fewer friends, and to play with younger children. During our evaluation, we noted that the patient had a thin, well-healed 1.5-cm scar on his forehead. Skull X rays revealed a 1.0-cm piece of shrapnel in his forehead. MRI revealed substantial loss of cortex in both frontal lobes. He showed steady improvement after information was given to the family and school regarding the nature of his brain injury and his special educational needs.

Case Example 2

A 34-year-old Hmong man presented with episodes of hyperventilation, palpitations, tachycardia, perspiration, chest pain, impaired mentation, and a sensation of impending doom. Cardiac and pulmonary assessments had been negative. These episodes were precipitated by the arrival in his local community of his former military commander, who had led a deep penetration into enemy-held territory more than a decade earlier. This commander had been lax regarding unit security, despite the fact that more than 200 men were involved in the maneuver. During an overnight bivouac several days into the march, the commander failed to set sentries or to send out small units to survey the local area. At dawn, the unit was surrounded and attacked; half of the unit was killed in the ambush. Despite a bullet wound to his buttocks, the patient was able to escape the field, carrying a comrade who had a leg fracture caused by a bullet. Survivors, pursued by the enemy, split up into small groups. During the flight, the patient left his friend on a ridge and went down to a valley stream for water. Hearing gunfire on the ridge, he returned and found that his comrade had been killed by the enemy.

When seen in our clinic, the patient was beset by a constant impulse to kill his former commander (an impulse he viewed as irrational and unacceptable), two to three panic attacks per day, and nightmares involving his dead friend. He responded well to a 3-month regimen of antidepressant medication and abreaction-integrative psychotherapy and counseling for missed bereavement of his deceased comrade.

Case Example 3

A 38-year-old Lao health care worker had been incarcerated in a prison camp in 1975 by the new Communist regime. Although psychologically demeaned, he was adequately nourished and not seriously harmed or physically threatened. However, several people in his camp were summarily executed for disrespect or disobedience toward their Lao guards. After 3 years of captivity, he led a successful escape involving several of his fellow prisoners. They all survived the several weeks' trek to the Mekong River, but one of his companions was shot in the head and killed as they came under fire while swimming the river.

On the anniversary of his comrade's death, he developed symptoms that initially included nightmares, sad-angry mood change, and severe headaches. These symptoms were treated in the refugee camp and later in the United States with minor opioids (e.g., codeine), which the patient began using routinely for minor symptoms. He was evaluated during his first year in the United States during an episode of this anniversary relapse. At that time he had PTSD and opioid dependence. He responded well to abrupt complete drug withdrawal, counseling for missed bereavement, and abreaction-integrative psychotherapy over a period of several weeks. During subsequent anniversaries, he developed less severe symptoms that responded to one or two psychotherapy sessions.

Case Example 4

A 42-year-old Hmong woman presented with inability to sleep alone in a darkened room at night. Although she had had this symptom for several years, her condition was exacerbated by the death of her husband several months earlier. She had recently become addicted to opium in an effort to relieve her fears, insomnia, and severe nightmares that involved the ghost or spirit of her deceased daughter. This daughter had died during a mortar attack on their village in Laos. As the patient and another woman were fleeing with their several children along a forest trail, a mortar round exploded nearby, injuring the daughter mortally and several others to a minor degree. The girl had massive injuries to her chest and abdomen, which caused organs to protrude. However, she was breathing and remained conscious. Mortar shells continued to explode around them, so the patient sent her remaining children with the other woman while she attempted to carry the 8-year-old child. This proved impossible in the mountainous terrain. The child, with mortal wounds, lost consciousness but continued to breathe. Unable to carry the child further and distraught at the separation from her other three children, the woman determined that the best alternative would be to bury her dying but still breathing child beneath a layer of rocks and dirt so that "the tigers would not eat her and she would have a proper burial." In the midst of keeping her other children alive during the subsequent flight through the countryside, she did not grieve this child. Over the years she kept the burial a secret.

At the time of evaluation, she manifested opioid dependence along with symptoms of major depressive disorder, PTSD, and phobia with panic. Following opioid withdrawal treatment, her major depressive disorder, PTSD, and phobia with panic persisted and became worse. Treatment next included treatment with antidepressant medication for her major depressive disorder and panic and then desensitization-type behavioral modification of her phobias of being in a darkened room by herself and sleeping in a room by herself. Grief counseling for her missed bereavement was instituted. After several weeks of intensive therapy, she was able to leave the hospital. In the outpatient department, abreaction-integrative psychotherapy was undertaken over a period of several months while she remained on antidepressant medication. She was followed over the subsequent year in a substance disorder program for refugees, through which her opioid-free rehabilitation and adjustment to American society were facilitated.

Problems with previous medical, psychological, and social assistance also occurred in this group, usually in association with failure to obtain a careful history of previous victimization. These problems were as follows:

- Both a pediatrician and a school psychologist had failed to elicit the trauma history or to recognize extensive frontal lobe damage in the 13-year-old Vietnamese boy.
- In their medical evaluation of the 34-year-old Hmong man, a cardiologist and a pulmonologist had failed to elicit the patient's trauma history or the precipitating event for his heart and breathing symptoms. In their reports, they made no mention of the bullet wound to his buttocks, despite a large tissue defect and extensive scarring.
- Physicians in a Thailand refugee camp and in an American clinic had treated the 38-year-old Lao man's headaches without eliciting data regarding the anniversary nature of his symptoms and their relationship to his incarceration, his role in planning the escape, and the death of his comrade during the escape.
- An internist had treated the 42-year-old Hmong woman for her insomnia with sedatives, without eliciting her trauma history or attempting to diagnose her several associated psychiatric conditions.

Demographics

These patients were several years younger than the patients in the previous group, having a mean age of 35.7 years (SD 13.5). Second, a higher-than-expected number of them were Hmong (28.7% of the Hmong patients in the study were in this group, and 12.6% of the patients of other ethnicities in the study were in this group). Third, the number of men in this group (43) was approximately twice the number of women (20). And fourth, fewer were widowed, separated, or divorced in this group (13 of 63) than in the previous group.

Clinical Characteristics

As in the previous group, mood disorder was the most prevalent diagnosis, occurring in 76% of patients. Psychoactive substance use disorders were present in 13% of cases. Psychosis not due to mood disorder (e.g., schizophrenia, drug-precipitated psychosis, schizophreniform psychosis) was present in 8%, although no such cases occurred in the previous group. PTSD diagnosed at the time of initial presentation was present in only 8%, although a few patients subsequently were found to have PTSD as their other conditions (e.g., psychosis, psychoactive substance use disorder) were treated successfully.

Medical conditions were slightly less common than in the previous group but were noted in 48% of cases. Some were related to injuries sustained during attack (e.g., amputation, brain injury, burns). Some somatic disorders that could be exacerbated by psychological factors were not directly related to trauma but did begin after the traumatic experiences (e.g., migraine, gastritis).

At the time of their initial evaluation, these patients showed a somewhat higher Axis V rating ("highest level of coping in the previous year") than did the previous group. Their mean score was 4.0, or "fair" (SD 1.0). Following treatment, most patients showed improvement on Axis V, with scores of 3 (or "good") to 2 (or "very good").

Treatment

Although most patients demonstrated good improvement, several patients failed to improve with treatment. These included four patients with psychoactive substance use disorders and four patients with one or another type of psychosis. Lack of cooperation with treatment regimens was present in most of these cases of treatment failure.

In addition, several patients had subsequent recurrences of their disorder, albeit in milder forms that required shorter courses of treatment.

For example, one Hmong combat veteran developed major depressive disorder and PTSD after he was laid off from work during a recession. Three years later he developed the same disorders when temporarily laid off. Whereas it required 22 visits and 6 months to treat his first episode successfully, his second episode resolved with four sessions over 1½ months.

Category Three:
Absence of Harm or Threat-of-Harm Experience

The largest number of refugees were in this category (207 or 72.4%).

Definition

These patients did not experience personal harm or threat of harm in the country of origin or during refugee flight out of the country into the country of refuge. Nonetheless, the fear of harm or threat was a major component in the decision to flee in most cases. Many patients in this category had relatives or friends who had been traumatized, either deliberately or impersonally.

As in the case of the patients in the previous two categories, these patients experienced loss of country, culture, and home. Many lost friends and relatives in Asia, and a few were victims of violence in the United States. However, none in this group were deliberately abused while in the hands of military or civilian authorities. None had been under attack during combat, experienced military attack on their communities, or been under attack during their escape from their home country. Still, their losses were extensive.

Discussion of Patients

Case Example 1

A 14-year-old Vietnamese boy was seen for inability to learn English, apathy, and social withdrawal. He was found also to have fatigue, hypersomnia, feelings of helplessness and worthlessness, headaches, loss of interest and enjoyment, and suicidal ideas. No cognitive deficits were noted. During his escape from Vietnam on a boat, both of his accompanying relatives (his father and an uncle) died of starvation. Placed with an American family, the patient had no contacts with other Vietnamese in the United States. He had no contacts with his family remaining in Vietnam and no notion of how they might be contacted. Diagnosed as having major depressive disorder and missed bereavement, he responded to antidepressant medication, bereavement counseling, being given information regarding methods to contact his family, and a milieu change that included placement with a Vietnamese family and attendance at a school with numerous Vietnamese adolescents.

Case Example 2

An 18-year-old Vietnamese man was seen with irascibility, inability to adjust to two previous American families, and academic failure. He had been in daily psychoanalytical treatment with a psychiatrist-analyst in another state for 6 months, with further deterioration during treatment. During assessment, he manifested intrusiveness, grandiosity, pressured speech, and inability to remain on one topic of conversation. He revealed that his family in Vietnam had paid for him to escape from Vietnam without other family members because the family feared that his taunting of Communist authorities and his antiauthoritarian attitudes and behaviors at school (beginning in midadolescence) were endangering the entire family. His foster family indicated that he ate voluminously (even when compared with their other teenage children), gained no weight, slept little, was constantly in motion, and seemed to pay no attention to authority.

A diagnosis of manic disorder was made, and lithium carbonate therapy was begun on an outpatient basis. Within several days, the patient's behavior at home and at school was within normal limits. However, for the first time he manifested sadness, expressed homesickness for Vietnam, and had some crying spells. These symptoms responded to grief counseling, supportive psychotherapy, and a discussion of plans regarding means for reuniting with his family. Over the next few years, he graduated from high school with superior grades, contacted his family, took a part-time job to send them money, entered the university (where he continued to receive superior grades), and managed to bring his parents and siblings to the United States on the Orderly Departure Program.

Case Example 3

A 19-year-old Hmong man had insidious onset of numerous cognitive and behavioral problems. These included paranoid ideas of others being against him, initiation of fights at school because of presumed slights against him, arguments with family members because of their presumed disrespect of him, a decrease in his grades, auditory hallucinations, and attempts to locate money and other valuable property that God presumably had sent to him. His family had survived the flight of Laos intact, and he had been educated in American grade school and high schools. Formerly, he had been an A student. There was no history of trauma, infectious disease, or victimization.

A diagnosis of schizophrenia was made, and he was hospitalized for a course of neuroleptic medication. After several rehospitalizations due to medication noncompliance, he eventually took antipsychotic medication as prescribed. His parents subsequently arranged his marriage to an unattractive but highly intelligent and competent Hmong woman, who supported the family with her job. They had three children, and the patient successfully adapted to acting as the family homemaker.

Case Example 4

A 37-year-old Hmong woman presented with major depressive disorder after several years in the United States. During the flight from Laos, she was separated from her husband. Subsequently, she spent a year in a Thai refugee camp with her four preschool children and a psychotic sister-in-law. Her father, a civil leader, was imprisoned and then died in a prison camp under mysterious circumstances. Upon reuniting with her husband in the United States, she had dealt with these earlier stressors and losses. However, the precipitating event for her current major depressive disorder was her husband's recent delusional disorder, which involved his firm belief that she was having sexual relations with literally scores of men, including several of his own relatives (despite much evidence to the contrary). Subjected to humiliations and beatings by her husband, she became depressed as she realized the nature of his condition, his resistance to treatment, and the family's powerlessness to deal with this situation in the American legal system. She responded well to supportive psychotherapy, a course of antidepressant medication, and separation from her husband.

As in the other two groups, some previous clinicians had overlooked history that was critical to understanding many cases. However, this was less often a problem in this group than in the other two groups, as demonstrated by the following:

- The 14-year-old bereaved Vietnamese boy was placed in a milieu that hampered the grieving of his recent losses as well as his sociocultural adjustment, resulting in a major depressive disorder.
- The 18-year-old Vietnamese man was misdiagnosed by a psychoanalyst as having an adjustment reaction, which had been treated with daily psychoanalytical sessions over several months without improvement. This resulted in his expulsions from two foster homes and, eventually, from a community that would not permit him to remain in school. He eventually did well when treated for mania. (Mania was not recognized by experienced American clinicians in several other cases, perhaps because of the moderation of behavioral components of mania among these patients, although their psychological manifestations were essentially similar to those of native-born American patients.)
- The 19-year-old Hmong man was rapidly and accurately diagnosed as having schizophrenia. However, poor compliance over a period of several months resulted in numerous family crises and rehospitalizations until the patient and family perceived the benefit of maintenance medication and of monitoring of his medication dosage and clinical condition.
- The 37-year-old Hmong woman sought early psychiatric consultation and was rapidly assessed and treated. Her course of treatment was short and her recovery was rapid and uneventful.

Reasons for the more timely treatment in this group probably include the following: a lower incidence of substance use disorders, a lower incidence of PTSD (which can complicate diagnosis and delay care), a lower incidence of traumatic brain injury, absence of care inappropriate for torture victims, greater trust in health and social resources, and more typical psychiatric clinical presentations.

Demographics

All ethnicities were equally represented. This group had the youngest mean age: 32.3 years (SD 14.3). Potentially pathogenic factors for the current disorders in the patients in this group included losses and stressors that did not involve military or governmental victimization, preexisting psychopathology developed in Asia, and onset of major mental illness with no apparent losses or stressors. Slightly more women were represented in this group (110 women vs. 97 men). Marital status was similar to that in the group exposed to impersonal violence.

Clinical Characteristics

Mood disorders were again the most prevalent psychiatric disorders, occurring in 72% of patients. PTSD at the time of initial assessment was infrequent, occurring in only one patient. Psychoactive substance use disorder was relatively infrequent compared with the other two groups (4%), whereas schizophrenia and other nonmood psychoses (such as schizophreniform psychosis and delusional disorder) were relatively frequent (11%).

Medical conditions were present in 57% of these cases, slightly more than in the group exposed to impersonal violence. These conditions included several life-threatening, nontraumatic conditions of a type not common in the other two groups (e.g., lung cancer, rheumatic heart disease, leprosy). Several patients had endocrine disorders (e.g., panhypopituitarism following postnatal hemorrhage in Asia, hyperthyroidism, hypothyroidism). Psychophysiological disorders such as asthma, eczema, allergic rhinitis, and migraine were common.

At the time of patients' initial evaluation, the Axis V rating "highest coping level in the previous year" was highest in this group, at 3.4 (between 3.0 or "good" and 4.0 or "fair").

Treatment

The majority of patients in this group did well in treatment. Treatment-resistant cases were relatively infrequent but qualitatively similar to those in the group exposed to impersonal violence.

Discussion

Ethnicity showed one major difference among these three groups of patients. Compared with non-Hmong patients in this group, the Hmong were considerably more apt to be impersonally traumatized by combat, village attacks, aerial assaults using toxic aerosols, and ambushes during refugee flight (29% of Hmong vs. 12% of non-Hmong patients, $\chi^2 =$ 19.67, $P < .001$). Conversely, the lowland Southeast Asians (i.e., Cambodians, Lao, Vietnamese, and ethnic Chinese) were more likely to have been tortured or deliberately traumatized while being held captive (12% of lowlanders vs. 2% of Hmong). This difference was a reflection of the high level of combat in the Laotian mountains and the frequent use of torture and terror as political weapons in lowland areas.

Average age also showed a difference among the three groups at $P < .005$ ($F = 5.93$), with victims of deliberate violence being the oldest, victims of impersonal violence being intermediate, and other refugees being the youngest. Males made up 63% of the group exposed to deliberate violence, 68% of the group exposed to impersonal violence, and 47% of the third group. An inordinate number of divorced, separated, and widowed patients were found among deliberately traumatized patients ($\chi^2 = 11.12$, $P < .005$). In sum, victims exposed to deliberate violence were more apt to be older men in leadership positions. The wives of some of these men were also deliberately traumatized but were allowed to live free after their husbands had been murdered or kept in prison. Among the victims of impersonal violence, many were younger male soldiers, although approximately one-third were women whose villages had been attacked or who had been attacked during refugee flight.

Among the 10 current cases of PTSD, 9 were related to previous refugee-related trauma and 1 case was related to recent trauma in the United States. The differences in percentages in each category (25% among victims of deliberate violence, 8% among victims of impersonal violence, and 0.5% among others) were statistically significant at $P < .001$ ($\chi^2 = 16.65$). The relatively lower incidence of PTSD in our sample compared with other samples of refugees could be due to differences in method. We used diagnoses made during the current evaluation rather than diagnoses made over patients' lifetimes. Use of the latter method would have increased the rate appreciably. We also did not include cases in which patients were not disabled or seriously discomforted by post-traumatic stress symptoms—which were frequent in this group. Examples included less-than-monthly nightmares, distress at watching a particular type of movie or television program, or anniversary symptoms that resolved spontaneously in hours or days and did not produce functional disability. In addition, we did not include cases in which such trauma-related symptoms ceased with treatment of the associated psychiatric condition and did not require additional treatment. Finally, we did not experience the kind of secondary-gain pressures encountered in other victimized-patient groups, for whom the PTSD diagnosis may provide monetary compensation. More impaired psychosocial coping was related to more severe victimization (at $P < .001$, $F = 10.98$), perhaps in part due to the presence of both PTSD and other associated psychiatric pathology, as well as to traumatic injuries in some patients.

Mood disorders (e.g., major depressive disorder, dysthymia, and bipolar disorder) were the most frequent diagnoses in all three groups. Of interest, three of the deliberately traumatized victims with a mood disorder had psychotic depression (of a total of 7 cases of psychotic depression in the total sample of 286 patients), suggesting that more severe mood disorders may prevail among torture victims. It appeared that psychoactive substance use disorders and organic mental disorders might show a trend for association with deliberate victimization, but a larger sample would be needed to test this adequately. Conversely, nonaffective psychoses (i.e., schizophrenia, delusional disorder, other nonaffective psychoses) were not particularly common among victims of deliberate violence. Axis III medical conditions were present in a large proportion of cases in all three categories. These conditions included posttraumatic disabilities (in the patients exposed to deliberate or impersonal violence), psychophysiological disorders (e.g., asthma, gastrointestinal conditions), tropical infections, substance-related disease, and degenerative conditions.

These findings indicate that histories and physical examinations regarding previous trauma are neglected by those serving refugee populations, including relocation workers, physicians (from pediatricians to internists to psychiatrists), and psychologists. Although overall rates of Axis III medical conditions did not differ among the three groups, sequelae of trauma were more frequent in the victimized groups. Average differences were demonstrated among the three groups with regard to gender (more male patients had been victimized), age (patients exposed to deliberate or impersonal violence were older than patients who were not exposed), marital status (more widowed, separated, and divorced patients had been deliberately victimized), PTSD diagnosis, and Axis V coping before treatment (poorer coping among those with more victimization).

Finally, this study demonstrates that refugee victims differ with regard to their previous victimization. Awareness concerning such differences can aid in allocating resources, in promoting awareness regarding victimization among refugee groups, and in decreasing ignorance and/or lack of relevant skills among clinicians who serve refugees. Such studies can also help us to oppose victimizers by bringing their activities to light and by restoring their victims to health.

References

Allodi F, Cowgill G: Ethical and psychiatric aspects of torture: a Canadian study. Can J Psychiatry 27:98–102, 1982

Allodi F, Stiasny S: Women as torture victims. Can J Psychiatry 35:144–148, 1990

American Psychiatric Association: Diagnostic and Statistical Manual of Mental Disorders, 3rd Edition. Washington, DC, American Psychiatric Association, 1980

American Psychiatric Association: Diagnostic and Statistical Manual of Mental Disorders, 3rd Edition, Revised. Washington, DC, American Psychiatric Association, 1987

American Psychiatric Association: Diagnostic and Statistical Manual of Mental Disorders, 4th Edition. Washington, DC, American Psychiatric Association, 1994

Amnesty International: Amnesty International Annual Report. London, Amnesty International Secretariat, 1994

Bacon KM: Population and power: preparing for change. Wall Street Journal, June 6, 1988, p 164

Cervantes RC, Salgado de Snyder VN, Padilla AM: Posttraumatic stress in immigrants from Central America and Mexico. Hospital and Community Psychiatry 40:615–619, 1989

Derogatis L: SCL-90-R Manual II. Towson, MD, Clinical Psychometric Research, 1983

Eberly RE, Engdahl BE: Prevalence of somatic and psychiatric disorders among former prisoners of war. Hospital and Community Psychiatry 42:807–813, 1991

Ford CV, Spauldy RC: The Pueblo incident: a comparison of factors relating to coping with extreme stress. Arch Gen Psychiatry 29:340–343, 1973

Goldfeld AE, Mollica RF, Pesavento BH, et al: The physical and psychological sequelae of torture: symptomatology and diagnosis. JAMA 259:2725–2729, 1988

Hamilton M: The assessment of anxiety states by rating. Br J Med Psychol 32:50–55, 1959

Hamilton M: A rating scale for depression. J Neurol Neurosurg Psychiatry 23:56–62, 1960

Helzer JE, Robins LN, McEvoy L: Posttraumatic stress disorder in the general population: findings of the Epidemiologic Catchment Area survey. N Engl J Med 317:1630–1634, 1987

Jensen TS, Genefke IK, Hydlebrandt N, et al: Cerebral atrophy in young torture victims (brief report). N Engl J Med 307:1341, 1982

Kinzie JD, Boehnlein JK, Leung PK, et al: The prevalence of posttraumatic stress disorder and its clinical significance among Southeast Asian refugees. Am J Psychiatry 147:913–917, 1990

Kluznik JC, Speed N, Van Valkenberg C, et al: Forty-year follow-up of United States prisoners of war. Am J Psychiatry 143:1443–1446, 1986

Kroll J, Habenicht M, MacKenzie T, et al.: Depression and posttraumatic stress disorder in Southeast Asian refugees. Am J Psychiatry 146:1592–1597, 1989

Lunde I, Rasmussen OV, Wagner G, et al: Sexual and pituitary-testicular function in torture victims. Arch Sex Behav 10:25–32, 1981

Mellman TA, Randolph CA, Brawman-Mintzer O, et al.: Phenomenology and course of psychiatric disorders associated with combat-related posttraumatic stress disorder. Am J Psychiatry 149:1568–1574, 1992

Mollica RF, Wyshak G, Lavelle J: The psychosocial impact of war trauma and torture on Southeast Asian refugees. Am J Psychiatry 144:1567–1572, 1987

Overall JE, Gorham DR: The Brief Psychiatric Rating Scale. Psychol Rep 10:799–812, 1962

Peters J, van Kammen D, van Kammen W, et al: Sleep disturbance and computerized axial tomographic scan findings in former prisoners of war. Compr Psychiatry 31:535–539, 1990

Rasmussen OV, Lunde I: Evaluation of investigation of 200 torture victims. Dan Med Bull 27:241–243, 1980

Rosen J, Reynolds CF, Yeager AL, et al.: Sleep disturbances in survivors of the Nazi Holocaust. Am J Psychiatry 148:62–72, 1991

Solkoff N, Gray P, Keill S: Which Vietnam veterans develop posttraumatic stress disorders? J Clin Psychol 42:686–698, 1986

Speed N, Engdahl B, Schwartz J, et al: Posttraumatic stress disorder as a consequence of the POW experience. J Nerv Ment Dis 177:147–153, 1989

Spitzer RL, Gibson M, Endicott J: Global Assessment Scale. New York, New York State Department of Mental Hygiene, 1973

Sutker PB, Winstead DK, Cahill ZH, et al: Cognitive deficits and psychopathology among former prisoners of war and combat veterans of the Korean conflict. Am J Psychiatry 148:67–72, 1991

Westermeyer JJ: Orientation to migrations and migrants, in Psychiatric Care of Migrants: A Clinical Guide. Washington, DC, American Psychiatric Press, 1989a, p 230

Westermeyer JJ: Public health aspects, in Mental Health for Refugees and Other Migrants: Social and Preventive Approaches. Springfield, IL, Chas C Thomas, 1989b, p 218

Westermeyer JJ, Wahmenholm K: Assessing the victimized psychiatric patient. Hospital and Community Psychiatry 40:245–249, 1989

Section III

Framework for Assessment and Treatment

CHAPTER 5

The Physician's Role in Assessment and Treatment of Torture Survivors

Federico Allodi, M.D., M.R.C.Psy.(U.K.), F.R.C.P.(C)

In 1975, Amnesty International, the prestigious human rights organization, published a report of a worldwide survey on torture as a practice of state control of political opposition (Amnesty International 1975). It was the first of its kind and included a fine essay on the medical and psychological aspects of torture. Subsequently, physicians associated with Amnesty International in Europe and North America reported their own observations on torture victims among groups of refugees from various parts of the world (Amnesty International 1977). There soon followed reports by other groups of physicians, affiliated with nongovernmental organizations, universities, and community clinics in countries in which refugees sought asylum or from which they fled (Allodi and Cowgill 1982; Cathcart et al. 1979; Cienfuegos and Monelli 1983).

Because of the United States' participation in the Vietnam War, many of the refugees who came to the United States came from Vietnam and other Southeast Asian countries (Mollica 1988). At the same time, observations on Vietnam War veterans gave rise to the development of the concept of posttraumatic stress disorder (PTSD), which was recognized as a diagnostic category by the American Psychiatric Association in DSM-III (American Psychiatric Association 1980). Historically, this concept was already implicit in Kardiner's "traumatic neuroses of war" (Kardiner 1947) and in the categories of combat exhaustion and gross stress reaction in the World Health Organization's *Manual of the International Classification of Diseases, Eighth Revision* (ICD-8) (World Health Organization 1969). By 1982, the psychological consequences of torture were proposed as a cluster of symptoms or a syndrome within the diagnostic category of PTSD (Allodi and Cowgill 1982). During the past decade, all major North American and European journals have published important articles on the subject of torture (Allodi 1991; Allodi and Stiasny 1990; Mollica et al. 1990; Ramsay et al. 1993; Reid and Strong 1988; Somnier and Genefke 1986) and a specialized journal, *The Journal of Traumatic Stress,* has carried articles on survivors of torture (Agger 1989; Agger and Jensen 1990).

In the 1990s, it is clear that the field of refugee trauma and, specifically, trauma of survivors of torture has become extensive and diffuse.

Major Issues in Medical Assessment and Care of Torture Survivors

Revision of the Concept of Posttraumatic Disorder

Although controversy continues about the merits and limitations of the concept of PTSD, this concept is a laudable effort to objectify and semiquantify a complex area of human experience. The concept has brought cohesiveness to a clinical picture that could have been easily muddled with an ill-assorted cluster of independent "syndromes" impossible to describe or compare according to any criteria or standards. It has also permitted more specific approaches to assessment and management, including organic, psychological, and social approaches. The diagnostic criteria (presence of a major stressor, hyperarousal, reexperiencing, and denial or avoidance) remain valid, although other symptoms present in victims of torture (somatoform, dissociative, and delusional symptoms) are being reported and their significance is being assessed (Kinzie and Boehnlein 1989; Ramsay et al. 1993). On the other hand, it is clear that only psychodynamic insights can directly approach issues of human consciousness and the disruption of psychic structures by the trauma (Benyakar et al. 1989).

Community Focus

Since the early 1960s, the community health concept has been supported by governments and by a large section of the public, including health professionals. Community health proposes a broader concept of health and illness, with emphasis on prevention, rehabilitation, and the social environment. However, the community of the 1990s is considerably different from that of past decades. The massive Asian, Caribbean, and Latin American migrations of the last decade have brought major changes to North American communities. There also have been gradual changes in the types and roles of the various professions and disciplines in the health care field, some of these changes still in the process of regulation. Rapid social change is a global phenomenon, and similar events, both in immigration and in other professional fields, have occurred on the European continent. Multicultural, racial, professional, gender, class, and generational issues and dynamics have acquired relevance and force.

Multiculturalism

As the result of the democratic acceptance of a pluralistic society, brought about by the technological revolution in communication and travel and by the development of the Third World, new concepts from cultural and social anthropology have been incorporated into medical vocabulary and practice. Most helpful are the concepts of culture, however it may be defined. These concepts include the distinction between traditional or premodern and modern cultures and between urban or industrial cultures, as well as the value of the individual rather than the family and community in modern society. The concept of explanatory models of health and illness, as part of the worldview or philosophy of a people, is essential in understanding treatment expectations and compliance of traditional people facing modern medical services (Kleinman 1980).

Multidisciplinary Context

The existence of other health care professionals in the health care field has always meant that the primary care physician and the psychiatrist work in an interdisciplinary environment. The 1950s, 1960s, and 1970s saw the appearance of psychologists, sociologists, counselors, therapists, and cultural anthropologists. Each one, directly or indirectly, has made important contributions to patient care and to medicine, especially when physicians were able to incorporate the new ideas and techniques into their own repertoire. In this regard, the "medical" model has proven resourceful and adaptable enough to become anything that physicians cared to conceive and practice on behalf of their patients' health and well-being. The 1980s saw the replacement of traditional hospital administrators by corporate organization managers. These new administrators have posed a special challenge: physicians need to become knowledgeable about the ideas and techniques of management and administration (including budget drafting and budget watching) if they are to retain their own identity and clinical independence in the service of their patients and their profession.

Psychotropic Medications

The use of tricyclic and tetracyclic antidepressants and the benzodiazepine sedatives in PTSD and the favorable results have been extensively reported (Schwartz 1990). No published report, however, has addressed the use of psychopharmacological agents for treating torture victims.

Other Treatment Modalities

Behavior, group, and art therapies; massage; physiotherapy; and expressive therapies have been used in treating survivors of torture (Agger and Jensen 1990; Allodi and Cowgill 1982; Fischman and Ross 1990). However, as with drug therapy, no evaluation of such interventions has been published so far.

Geopolitical Changes

The international scene has become ever more complex and changeable. It continues to create refugees and victims of man-made trauma including war, genocide, terrorism, deportation, concentration camp experience, massive rape, and torture (Westermeyer 1989). The instability of the world's demographic, socioeconomic, and political situation has increased the number of international refugees, now 20 million, and presents new scenarios of trauma. It challenges humanitarian groups and concerned physicians involved in reporting human rights violations and in caring for victims. As a rule, sovereign states openly deny any accusations of torture committed by their own security apparatus or by their allies or friendly governments, whereas they are ready to denounce with alacrity the actions of their enemies and unfriendly nations. The idea of a double standard in human rights tests the ethical position of physicians in their own consciences and, at times, in their practices. There is little doubt that this double standard plays a part in the dynamics of countertransference (Gorkin 1986) and/or research and publication priorities.

As a consequence of the aforementioned developments, physicians, including psychiatrists, need to define their own roles and tasks as clearly as possible.

Assessment: Principles and Practice

The primary function of a physician in any society is to be a diagnostician and healer of illness and health problems in an individual, family, or community. The history given by the patient or relatives and friends and the observations made by the physician in the first interview or interviews are still the basic sources of information that will dictate the diagnostic and treatment conclusions. The problem for which the physician is consulted must be defined as clearly as possible. In the case of people from different cultures (e.g., refugees), the history must be allowed to be in the form of a narrative, that is, an expression of the patient's experience in terms of his or her own worldview, explanations of causes of illness, and expectations of services. The narrative also permits the physician to accept the personal experience of the patient and to regard the patient as a person rather than as a source of data needed to arrive at a diagnostic category. Rape and torture are major traumas, often accounting for a full-blown PTSD, but from the patient's perspective, they are unique and deeply personal experiences that in some way must be expressed and shared (Kleinman 1988).

Caution must be exercised in taking the history of the trauma (be it rape, torture, or the witnessing of the death or suffering of friends and loved ones) on two accounts. First, not everything can be expressed; no language in any culture can express adequately a particular traumatic experience. The novelist Joseph Conrad visited the Congo Free State, ruled by King Leopold II of Belgium, who caused the death of unnamed millions of native Congolese between 1885 and 1908. In Conrad's novel *Heart of Darkness,* the character Captain Kurtz could say only: "The horror, the horror . . . " These words were later repeated about the Vietnam War in the movie *Apocalypse Now.* By allowing the patient his or her own narrative and expression of the experience, sometimes only in silence and tears, the physician can respect the depth of suffering and the limits of the language.

The second caution on history taking is that the telling of the story of the trauma is nearly as painful as the experience of the trauma. Some images of trauma are so painful that it will be many years before they can be recalled without a throb of that pain. It is natural to avoid repeating the story or even to deny that the trauma ever happened. The mechanism of denial is also very effective in protecting the victim from the consequences of confronting the brutal and unacceptable reality. The following story was given to me, while I was on a consulting visit to a Central American country in July 1991, by an official of a human rights organization. He said:

> I had the sorry task of informing a mother that the body of her 24-year-old son had been found after 2 months' disappearance and of asking her to come to the morgue to identify him. I knew the young man, and when the body was shown to us, of course I recognized him immediately. The mother, to my surprise, said quite definitely and calmly: "This is not my boy. No, it is not." I did not know what to say, for I knew it was her son. I said nothing and we went out into the street. We walked for a while and then the woman said: "Let us go back and take a second look, just in case I made a mistake." We did go back to the morgue, drew out again the cool box where the body was contained, and looked at him. The mother recognized her son and in tears and laments she collapsed to the ground.

Clearly, the mechanism of denial initially protected the woman from severe psychological suffering and physiological distress. The paradoxical nature of denial and avoidance are common experiences in the analytical therapy of repressed memories and mental contents. The repressed experience is the central theme, but the attention actively moves around it without directly focusing on it, like the eyes of an actor in front of the camera: the lens must be foremost in the actor's mind for the actor to be able to avoid and ignore it.

After taking the history of the presenting problem and the experience of trauma, the physician must then elicit the symptoms of distress or ill health; describe and measure any lasting scars or other physical sequelae; and record the details of dates and places of the trauma and the names of those people or organizations responsible or involved. The extent to which this is possible in a first interview depends on the quality of the patient-doctor relationship and, specifically, on the degree of trust that has been established.

In few other areas of medical practice is the relationship of trust more important and possibly more difficult than in examining and treating victims of torture. The essential damage of torture is located in the mental representation of the "other," as opposed and necessarily linked to the "self." The other is to be understood also as the primordial structure or relationship with other people, initiated by the interaction between the mother and the infant, internalized in the core of the mind as part of the stable, cohesive, worthy, and autonomous self. It is equivalent to the psychoanalytical concept of "object relations" (meaning personal relations with people or emotionally meaningful objects or places) (Hamilton 1992). Only when the other is apprehended in the conscious mind will it gain a separate reality or existence and become part of the realm of consciousness and the conscious life of the self, which is the center of psychological life. The first interview is an opportunity for the doctor to gain access to the damaged structure of the other and, through treatment, to begin the restoration of the damaged self.

The Medicolegal Assessment

A special form of consultation is often required of primary care physicians or psychiatrists for medicolegal purposes. The resulting report may be of considerable importance for providing evidence to support a claim for refugee status. Secondarily, it may provide an opportunity to restore the social image of the person so badly tarnished by the trauma. In addition, it is also possible that, in the future, the report may be used as evidence in reparation claims against guilty governments or agents. Furthermore, such reports, while preserving anonymity, have provided the basic data and material for medical and human rights reports and publications that have done so much in the past two decades to fight the epidemic of torture. In many countries, both north and south of the equator, these reports grew out of the collaboration between doctors and lawyers, often at an informal and ad hoc level, and later formed the basis for some of the earliest community clinics and centers for torture victims (Jaranson 1995). The issues that follow are those generally to be considered in these medical reports.

Establishment of Link Between Trauma of Torture and Symptoms of Distress

It is helpful to describe succinctly the trauma endured, if possible with dates, places, and names; the early symptoms and their evolution; treatment received, if any, and when and where it was received; and, finally, the current symptoms. The diagnosis should be established with reference to the list of criteria for PTSD in DSM-IV (American Psychiatric Association 1994). DSM-IV has also listed a condition, acute stress disorder, that was not previously listed in DSM-III-R (American Psychiatric Association 1987) but that was included in ICD-9 (World Health Organization 1977) and ICD-10 (World Health Organization 1992) as acute stress reaction. Acute stress disorder has the same list of criteria as PTSD but is differentiated from it by the addition to the list of acute dissociative symptoms and the specific criterion of having less than 1 month's duration. This category includes combat fatigue. Alternatively, if the needed criteria for PTSD are not met, any other diagnosis unrelated to it or related to it as a complication should be established. Often major depressive disorder, or reactive depressive disorder consequent to trauma, as well as psychotic episodes, has been diagnosed in a proportion of cases following trauma.

Credibility or Reliability of Information Given by Victim

A statement should be made on the internal congruence of the information given, that is, on the medical correspondence or fit between the trauma and the clinical reaction or symptoms and signs observed. Most commonly, the lasting sequelae shown by survivors of torture are psychological, but even in these cases they are not always specific, with the exception of some phobias and nightmares and flashbacks. Often one sees physical damage and scars of torture, which should be described or photographed and produced as objective evidence. These physical signs include cigarette burns; unreduced fractures of fingers; circular scars on the wrists or ankles from handcuffs, leg irons, or ropes; and multiple linear scars from whipping and lacerations on the back or buttocks. Further hard evidence can be obtained through X rays in cases of allegations of fractures or severe blows to the body, limbs, or head. These searches for evidence often turn out to be fruitless, however, because torture is designed with the aim of leaving no such traces or the character of the trauma may be nonspecific.

The reliability of the history can be strengthened by its external coherence or logic, that is, by its fitting into the context of torture in that particular time and country. The physician should be familiar with the reports of Amnesty International or other reputable nongovernmental organizations or human rights groups, so that he or she can make a judgment about the probability of such events occurring in that country to the patient. The status, occupation, and sociopolitical activities of the victim and any media, personal documentation, or hospital records may add external evidence. Gathering this type of evidence is strictly the responsibility of the patient and not of the physician, but advising the victim to secure that evidence may strengthen the patient-doctor relationship and, in any case, falls within the traditional role of the physician of counseling the suffering and the needy.

Prognostic Statements

The motivation of the governments giving asylum to survivors of torture, other violent persecution, and man-made trauma is a mixture of humanitarianism and self-interest. It is no surprise that these governments should be interested in whether the new arrivals are going to be a burden to the host community. From the medical and psychological point of view, the answers cannot be definite, because there are no long-term follow-up studies using sound methodology. Brief follow-up studies have been conducted mostly on populations in treatment and naturally show a bias through selecting cases with poor outcome and in need of treatment. Some exceptions can be found in studies of groups of refugee children, orphaned or with their parents, arriving in countries such as Canada, the United

States, and Australia. These studies reported that outcomes were favorable when public attitudes were welcoming and a network of social support were brought to help the children and their families (Allodi 1989; Krupinski 1986; Sokoloff et al. 1984).

The long-term outcome of the survivors of those experiences is uncertain. Occasionally clinicians see adults who, having recovered from major traumas in their early childhood, perform successfully as parents and working people, yet, after a precipitating event or a minor trauma 20 or 30 years later, reexperience the early trauma, with catastrophic results.

As for individuals who were exposed to torture as adults, it is common experience among clinicians that in the majority of cases, after the acute stages, the psychological symptoms of PTSD do not cause social or occupational disability. The miscellaneous symptoms of depression, suspiciousness, or fleeting paranoid ideas also respond favorably to psychopharmacological and psychotherapeutic treatment. Somatoform and dissociative symptoms appear when there has been a complicating life event in the country of exile (difficulties in obtaining refugee status; occupational, family, or political problems; illnesses; financial stresses). The symptoms may have a secondary advantage in that they may cause the patient to seek help for the aforementioned complicating events.

Alcohol abuse and other drug abuse often have been seen as coping mechanisms in youth who come from societies in which drugs are available and substance use is condoned by the culture. Addiction to trauma experiences as a means of coping, reported in Vietnam War veterans with PTSD (Solursh 1989), has not been reported in refugee survivors of torture but may explain in part the reports of drug and alcohol abuse, behavior disorders, and conflict with the law among refugees.

As an example of trauma addiction, a Central American cinematographer and survivor of torture gave a history of a posttraumatic career in which he volunteered and found himself repeatedly in the major trouble spots of the world (Lebanon, Iraq, Gaza and the West Bank, Bosnia-Herzegovina). He had been addicted to trauma experiences since his torture and admitted, "I miss the danger, the excitement, life at the brink. I love the rush. I want to identify myself with the people that are hurt and suffering."

The prognosis for the majority of these cases in treatment is fair, provided that adequate or comprehensive services and mechanisms for acculturation are available. At an inner psychological or existential level, the experience of torture, like any other massive trauma, is never forgotten and sometimes never compensated. The literature on the Jewish Holocaust amply demonstrates that, in many instances, the psyche has been too deeply wounded to reconstitute itself, and the damage and the suffering are permanent: "once a victim, always a victim." Personal experience and knowledge of the professional literature on this subject may enable the primary care physician and the psychiatrist to offer expert opinions on the probabilities of recovery from disability and maladaptation for a particular survivor.

Treatment

In the primary role of healer and as a consultant on treatment methods for torture survivors, psychiatrists and other physicians must have clear principles that will enhance the chances of effectively treating torture survivors: a holistic approach, a comprehensive concept of health and illness, and a dynamic understanding of trauma and recovery.

The concept of body-mind dualism has been helpful at a theoretical level and for abstract description and communication of patient problems. However, the medical and the psychological cannot be dissociated; they are one and the same and complementary. The patient experiences the trauma as a whole, and the doctor, who understands and empathizes with the patient's experiences, also experiences the problem as a whole. The doctor possesses concepts and treatment techniques for the body and mind but, in the dynamism of the patient-doctor relationship, does not perceive them as separate. It is the patient-doctor relationship that integrates the biological and the psychological in the process of care. Without this relationship, also called *therapeutic alliance, working alliance,* or *transference,* there may be no therapy or care.

The holistic approach is even more relevant for patients from traditional cultures in which worldviews and concepts of health and illness do not distinguish between psychological and physiological processes. The supernatural often is considered the cause of the good health or the illness of a person or community. In these cases, the acceptance by the physician of the patient experience integrates the soma and the psyche.

A conceptual model of therapy (Figure 5–1) accounts for essential

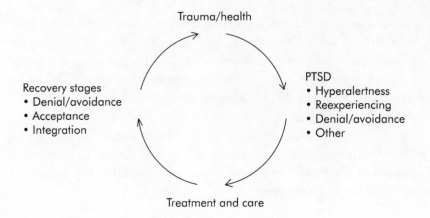

Trauma/health

Recovery stages
• Denial/avoidance
• Acceptance
• Integration

PTSD
• Hyperalertness
• Reexperiencing
• Denial/avoidance
• Other

Treatment and care

Treatment

Stage I: organic therapy: supportive, empathic
• Rest, medication, occupational/physiotherapy

Stage II: dynamic therapy
Surface level
• Abreactive, expressive
• Explanatory
• Cognitive coping
Depth level
• Personality/defenses discussion
• Analytical/self orientation (transference analysis)

Figure 5–1.   Trauma and recovery: a dynamic conceptual model.

observations and processes. When the model is used to describe therapy for trauma, the elements of the model are 1) health as a state of harmony or balance, given that all organisms tend to retain and return to that state of balance; 2) trauma as the agent disrupting the balance; 3) a posttraumatic state of varying degrees of disorganization, with signs and symptoms of strain, distress, or disorder, specifically PTSD; 4) treatment intervention and care; and 5) ideally, a stage of recovery and return to health. There are a number of models in the current literature, and most of them describe similar posttraumatic behavior and stages of recovery. In the recovery process, the victim goes through the phases of denial and avoidance, recalling, abreaction and acceptance, and, finally, integration or reconstruction of the history and meaning of the trauma (Herman 1992). Each stage requires appropriate therapist behavior and intervention. Whether the patient is a survivor of the Jewish Holocaust, child abuse, combat stress reactions, or torture, the stages of recovery and the principles of intervention are the same (Fogelman 1988; Noy 1991).

Most victims of torture and other violent persecutions have good pretrauma adjustment and healthy personalities. It is safe to assume that the natural tendency of the organism to heal itself is quite strong. The physician limits his or her role so that he or she is merely helping nature take its course. Immediately after the trauma and in the acute stages, all symptoms of PTSD are prevalent among those who have endured severe trauma; this was the case with Latin American and Southeast Asian refugees coming to North America in the late 1970s and early 1980s. First, organic forms of therapy (rest, sedatives, antidepressants, and sympathetic support and listening) are indicated and effective. Subsequently, dynamic methods are instituted. Victims requiring psychotherapy are provided short-term, intermediate, or profound therapy, as appropriate.

Short-term therapy consists of sympathetic listening as well as discussions and explanations of problems specifically linking the trauma with the present symptoms. At an intermediate level, therapy involves discussions of personality and defense or coping mechanisms as factors in the reaction to trauma. Finally, at a more profound level, patient and therapist travel to regions of the patient's psyche of which the patient is not yet conscious. In this joint venture, early childhood trauma and its personality consequences are reexamined and meaning is brought to the present posttraumatic conflicts.

The experience of torture, like that of any other painful trauma, is repressed and avoided, banished from clear consciousness. In this twilight or dark existence, it acts like a toxin, a festering wound. The image of the other is damaged and damages any possible relationship with other people, in particular those who, like doctors, may come close to the area where the trauma is hidden. In a relationship of trust or positive transference, the doctor tries to make a link with the undamaged portions of that self and related early positive experiences. In doing so, the physician may create the possibility of listening to or witnessing the reenactment of the trauma either in tears and silence or in narrative. Later, patient and physician, as companions, may explore and absorb the unconscious aspects of the trauma into a conscious world that, integrated, will strengthen the survivor's life and self. Where there were fear to remember and silence, there can be memory, a history, explanations, understanding, and trust. The self can appropriate and enrich itself with the traumatic experience.

In a case of good posttraumatic outcome, one patient said, "Many good things happened to me after the trauma. I learned a lot. Now I'm not so naive or idealistic." Another patient actively involved in human rights reported, "I'm having a good time."

On the other hand, some patients have difficulty integrating the impact of trauma. A man in his 30s experienced lengthy imprisonment and severe torture while he was in his late teens and a student leader. His mind was in a constant emotional and cognitive turmoil. This turmoil warped the perception of his social reality, as well as the transference situation with the therapist and with his employer, a mature, compassionate, and intelligent woman. Referring to the struggle with his employer and in therapy, he said, "Nobody has broken me: not my father, not my torturers, not anybody else." His father had been abusive, and the trauma of torture further deepened the wound in the son's heroic and narcissistic self. He saw little value in other experiences, both in his childhood and in his present situation, except for his own rigid and narcissistic defenses. Feeling superior to experiencing anger and resentment, incapable of compassion for himself or love for another person, he was unable to accept the reality of his situation and relate to it accordingly. His self lacked the attributes of integration: wholeness, continuity, and autonomy. He interrupted therapy. It is hoped that therapy can continue and can help him to develop more acceptance of those experiences and of himself.

Community Consultation

Physicians moving into the community of the 1990s as consultants or as members of an interdisciplinary team must be ready to recognize the community's nature and dynamics; those who ignore them do so at their own peril.

Even when the physician's role is described as consulting, in fact it is a collaborative function in a multidisciplinary context. The concept of *team,* so popular in the heady 1960s, is not much in favor these days. The most acceptable and productive concept is the social network of support. This refers to the system of social relationships and institutions that constitute the adaptive resources available to an individual, family, or community. The network has an informal or natural sector, such as family, friends, and neighbors, and a formal or professional sector, to which the health, social, legal, and judiciary institutions and agencies belong. The completeness and supportiveness of a network is a reflection of the degree of organization and strength of a community. In the mental health field, this network is considered a most significant factor in the recovery from illness; and, in the case of refugees, it is the emotional support qualities of the network that are specifically associated with favorable posttraumatic outcome (Fuch 1991). In the field of refugee trauma, physicians would function within the formal health sector and have regular contacts with the social, governmental, and other institutions and agencies of the network.

As a consultant or member of a collaborative group in the network of services for refugees and torture victims, the primary care physician or psychiatrist can contribute by means of the following:

- Designing and operating an intake or triage system for refugees (among whom there are likely to be survivors of torture), in refugee camps, residences, centers, or clinics.
- Advising on the institution and design of protocols, brief screening instruments, and criteria for referral of those refugees or survivors who are distressed and in need of medical or psychiatric consultation and care: the suicidal, potentially violent, psychotic, or persistently distressed.
- Participating in the supervision of and training programs for intake workers, counselors, medical students, and psychiatric residents, as well as other medical colleagues and psychiatrists who may require such services. (Unfortunately, there is no single adequate manual for training counselors and therapists working with survivors of torture. The main reason for this is that the recipients of training, the survivors themselves, and the context of therapy can be widely divergent. Health workers in refugee camps in Pakistan, at the Thai-Cambodian border, or Somalia face very different problems than do counselors and workers in Sweden, Canada, the United Kingdom, and the United States. Besides problems of inconsistent material and technical and human resources,

there exist problems of cultural disparity between counselors and refugees or survivors. Such problems also exist between the counselors or users of those manuals and the writers, who may come from developing countries but who have been trained in the modern Western world. The World Health Organization, the International Red Cross, and some European and American centers have made laudable attempts to meet the demand.)

- Participating in the design of data collection systems and research projects. Such participation includes outlining research priorities, selecting and drafting appropriate scales and questionnaires, analyzing data, and interpreting and directing research. Evaluation of the effectiveness of various treatment modalities and programs is sorely lacking, but it is, in fact, part of the responsibility of being a physician.

- Participating in the planning, organization, and managing or directing of agencies or institutions involved in the care and support of traumatized refugees and survivors of torture or participating in primary prevention programs, by promoting the links between medicine or health and human rights. The essential criterion for participation in any of these organizations or agencies, governmental or nongovernmental, is the compatibility of the objectives and means of operation of such organizations or projects with medical ethics, which will require that physicians act with complete independence of judgment and action in clinical matters and on behalf of patients and survivors of torture.

References

Agger I: Sexual torture of political prisoners: an overview. J Trauma Stress 2:305–318, 1989

Agger I, Jensen B: Testimony as ritual and evidence in psychotherapy for political refugees. J Trauma Stress 3:115–130, 1990

Allodi F: The children of victims of political persecution and torture: a psychological study of a Latin American refugee community. International Journal of Mental Health 18:3–15, 1989

Allodi F: Assessment and treatment of torture victims: a critical review. J Nerv Ment Dis 179:4–11, 1991

Allodi F, Cowgill G: Ethical and psychiatric aspects of torture: a Canadian study. Can J Psychiatry 27:98–102, 1982

Allodi F, Stiasny S: Women as torture victims. Can J Psychiatry 35:144–148, 1990

American Psychiatric Association: Diagnostic and Statistical Manual of Mental Disorders, 3rd Edition. Washington, DC, American Psychiatric Association, 1980

American Psychiatric Association: Diagnostic and Statistical Manual of Mental Disorders, 3rd Edition, Revised. Washington, DC, American Psychiatric Association, 1987

American Psychiatric Association: Diagnostic and Statistical Manual of Mental Disorders, 4th Edition. Washington, DC, American Psychiatric Association, 1994

Amnesty International: Report on Torture, Revised. London, Amnesty International Publications, 1975

Amnesty International. Evidence of Torture: Studies by the Amnesty International Danish Medical Group. London, Amnesty International Publications, 1977

Benyakar M, Kutz I, Dasberg H, et al: The collapse of a structure: a structural approach to trauma. J Trauma Stress 2:431–449, 1989

Cathcart IM, Berger P, Knazan B: Medical examination of torture victims applying for refugee status. Can Med Assoc J 121:179–184, 1979

Cienfuegos AJ, Monelli C: The testimony of political repression as a therapeutic instrument. Am J Orthopsychiatry 53:43–51, 1983

Fischman Y, Ross J: Group treatment of exiled survivors of torture. Am J Orthopsychiatry 60:135–142, 1990

Fogelman E: Therapeutic alternatives for Holocaust survivors and the second generation, in The Psychological Perspectives of the Holocaust and of Its Aftermath. Edited by Braham RL. New York, Columbia University Press, 1988

Fuch L: Factors affecting level of happiness among Southeast Asian refugee women in Saskatoon, in Immigrants and Refugees in Canada: A Natural Perspective on Ethnicity, Multiculturalism and Cross-Cultural Adjustment. Edited by Sharna SP. Toronto, Basic Books, 1991, pp 147–158

Gorkin M: Countertransference in cross-cultural psychotherapy. The example of Jewish therapist and Arab patient. Psychiatry 49:69–79, 1986

Hamilton NG: Self and Others: Object Relations Theory and Practice. Northvale, NJ, Jason Aronson, 1992

Herman JL: Trauma and Recovery. New York, Basic Books, 1992

Jaranson J: Governmental torture: status of the rehabilitation movement. Transcultural Psychiatric Research Review 32:253–286, 1995

Kardiner A: The Traumatic Neuroses of War. New York: Hoeber, 1947

Kinzie DJ, Boehnlein JJ: Posttraumatic psychosis among Cambodian refugees. J Trauma Stress 2:185–198, 1989

Kleinman A: Patients and Healers in the Context of Culture: An Explanation of the Borderland Between Anthropology, Medicine and Psychiatry. Berkeley, CA, University of California Press, 1980, pp 83–84

Kleinman AC: The Illness Narrative: Suffering, Healing and the Human Condition. New York, Basic Books, 1988

Krupinski J: Summary, in The Price of Freedom Among Indochinese refugees in Australia. Edited by Krupinsky J, Burrows G. Sydney, Australia, Pergamon Press, 1986, pp 232–243

Mollica R: The trauma story: the psychiatric care of refugee survivors of violence and torture, in Posttraumatic Therapy and Victims of Violence. Edited by Ochberg FM. New York, Brunner/Mazel, 1988

Mollica R, Wyshak G, Lavelle J, et al: Assessing symptom change in Southeast Asian refugee survivors of mass violence and torture. Am J Psychiatry 147:83–88, 1990

Noy S: Combat stress reactions, in Handbook of Military Psychology. Edited by Gal R, Mangelsdorff AD. New York, Wiley, 1991

Ramsay R, Gorst-Unsworth C, Turner S: Psychiatric morbidity in survivors of organized state violence including torture: a retrospective series. Br J Psychiatry 162:55–59, 1993

Reid JC, Strong T: Rehabilitation of refugee victims of torture and trauma: principles of service provision in New South Wales. Med J Aust 148:340–346, 1988

Schwartz LS: Biopsychosocial treatment approach to posttraumatic stress disorder. J Trauma Stress 3:221–238, 1990

Sokoloff BZ, Carlin JE, Pram H, et al: Five-year follow-up of Vietnamese refugee children in the United States. Part I. Clin Pediatr (Phila) 23:565–570, 1984

Solursh LP: Combat addiction: overview of implications in symptoms maintenance and treatment planning. J Trauma Stress 2:251–462, 1989

Somnier FE, Genefke IK: Psychotherapy for victims of torture. Br J Psychiatry 149:323–329, 1986

Westermeyer J: Cross-cultural care for PTSD: research, training and service needs for the future. J Trauma Stress 2:515–536, 1989

World Health Organization. Manual of the International Classification of Diseases, Eighth Revision (ICD-8). Geneva, World Health Organization, 1969

World Health Organization. Manual of the International Classification of Diseases, Injuries and Causes of Death, Ninth Revision (ICD-9). Geneva, World Health Organization, 1977

World Health Organization. The ICD-10 Classification of Mental and Behavioural Disorders: Clinical Descriptions and Diagnostic Guidelines. Geneva, World Health Organization, 1992

CHAPTER 6

How Medical Assessment of Victims of Torture Relates to Psychiatric Care

Neal R. Holtan, M.D., M.P.H., F.A.C.P.

A story of courage and healing by a doctor who was a prisoner in a concentration camp is told by Robert Lifton:

> A Jewish doctor who survived Auschwitz incarceration told me his story, and became my friend. He described how, at a certain point, he and a few other prisoner doctors were overwhelmed with moribund patients, with suffering people clamoring for relief. They did what they could, dispensed the few aspirin they had, but made a point in the process of offering a few words of reassurance and hope. He found, almost to his surprise, that his words had effect, that "in that situation it really helped." He concluded that by maintaining one's determination to try to heal, even under the most extreme conditions, "I was impressed with how much one could do." (Lifton 1986, p. 504)

This humbling example can serve as a starting point for the physician caring for a victim of torture. Once the torture survivor has come to a developed country, a physician may still offer primarily the simple but effective things available to the doctor in Auschwitz—relief from pain and "reassurance and hope."

Medical Examination of Survivors

Most of the patients at the Center for Victims of Torture (CVT) have come to Minneapolis as visitors or aliens without documents, seeking political asylum. They need the results of a medical examination to support their case for the granting of asylum. Although their medical problems are comparable to those of refugees to the United States, visitors and aliens differ from refugees in that they have not gone through the processes of the Immigration and Naturalization Service of the Justice Department and have not had routine medical examinations or screening for infectious disease.

In the medical interview and examination at CVT, the physician assesses the patient's physical health; psychiatric assessment and, if needed, treatment follow this initial assessment. The medical assessment includes the following components: a medical history, a physical examination, a skin test for tuberculosis, a vision and hearing screen, a dental evaluation, stool tests for ova and parasites, urinalysis, a serological test for syphilis, thyroid function tests, and a fasting lipid profile. In some cases, parts of this basic medical assessment have already been completed at another health care facility, but experience has shown that it is necessary to obtain copies of records from other medical encounters for review. Often other physicians are unfamiliar with the health problems of torture survivors and do not complete all components of the assessment.

The medical assessment sets the stage for psychological treatment. In particular, the primary care physician tries to control distressing and distracting physical symptoms so that the patient may be responsive to counseling, psychotherapy, and psychoactive medication (Chester and Holtan 1992). Besides identifying chronic medical conditions, the physician can encourage the patient to be physically active and to participate in social interactions. The medical assessment offers the physician the opportunity to promote the patient's acceptance of the need for psychological help and to lay groundwork for the therapeutic relationship.

Common Medical Findings

Patients who have been tortured may display severe psychological disorders such as delayed posttraumatic stress disorder (PTSD) and major depression (Herman 1992; Somnier et al. 1992). Torture victims often describe physical rather than psychological symptoms of their psychiatric disorders. For example, symptoms of PTSD, such as fatigue and lack of connection with surroundings, and symptoms of depression, such as insomnia, loss of libido, and poor appetite, may be strongly linked by the patient to old physical injuries, scars, or deformities due to the torture.

Pain—in the head, chest, abdomen, or back—is most often the primary initial complaint and concern of torture victims. Comparable complaints of severe pain offered in traditional settings by patients who have not experienced torture demand prompt physical evaluation, including the use of invasive diagnostic procedures. In patients who have been tortured, however, a slower, more deliberate, and less invasive approach works better because the pain may be a manifestation of a primary psychiatric problem.

Psychosomatic pain, if not addressed and treated when it occurs, can recur months and years after torture. Sometimes the pain relates to specific torture such as beating on the head, electrical torture of the chest or heart, or blows to the abdomen. Chronic low back pain, a symptom found in a large majority of torture victims evaluated in Denmark and elsewhere, occurs independently of the type of torture suffered (Skylv 1992). It does not correlate with trauma to the back, with hanging by the limbs, or with other abuse that might be expected to stress the back; rather, it may be analogous to a tension headache.

Physical signs result from various forms of torture (Basoglu 1993; Skylv 1992). Scars from beatings, whippings, and burns with cigarettes or hot objects; from searing with acid; and from cuts by knives and bayonets provide confirmation for survivors' reported histories. Scars can also result from deep abrasions caused by shackles and bindings. Other physical sequelae of torture may include fractures of long bones (now healed), damaged teeth, and punctured eardrums. A unique sequela of electrical torture is the picaña scar, where electricity was applied to the skin (Danielsen and Berger 1981). Falanga, a form of torture involving beating of the soles of the feet, can cause deformity and chronic disability of the feet (Skylv 1993).

For a majority of patients, pain and other psychological symptoms abate after a careful medical examination, a few appropriate tests, and reassurance from the physician that the brain, heart, and other organs are functioning well and have not been permanently harmed. Patients who do not improve with reassurance require analgesics or other treatments. Nonspecific symptoms, such as fatigue, cannot be ascribed to depression unless common medical causes have been ruled out. A 36-year-old man who had been tortured by being choked and by blows to the neck presented in Minneapolis with depression as a chief complaint. He had a neck scar that he claimed was a repaired laceration. On testing, he was found to have profound hypothyroidism. Another example of a medical disease masquerading as a psychological symptom in a torture victim in Minneapolis is hyperaldosteronism causing labile hypertension and a sensation of general malaise, labeled by the patient as anxiety.

Either the primary care physician or the psychiatrist can document the history of torture, the methods used, the injuries received, and any physical signs consistent with the history. Both can document psychiatric symptoms, the history of psychological trauma, and the patient's appearance, speech, mannerisms, mood, affect, and other aspects of mental status. This combined physical and psychological documentation provides the basis for the medical care plan; it is also the best way to support the patient's application for political asylum. The case is strengthened when the physician and the psychiatrist independently make similar observations regarding the patient's physical and psychological health.

Cross-Cultural Medical Assessment

Assessing and treating torture victims in developed countries requires practicing medicine across linguistic and cultural barriers (Morris and Silove 1992). Issues involved in the use of interpreters in health care are complex and beyond the scope of this chapter. Even when there is no language barrier or when the physician and the patient are able to communicate sufficiently, major cultural differences between the physician and the foreign-born patient are certain to exist.

As a complex form of human behavior, even torture has its cultural relativity, differing from one society to another in meaning and interpretation. When some patients are asked directly about torture, they may not label their past abuse as torture. For example, in some Middle Eastern countries, beatings by guards in a prison are viewed by the prisoners as a part of everyday life and not necessarily as torture. In some countries of the Far East, many people accept political torture as a punishment for failings in this life or in past ones.

Some health providers fear that torture victims may be unduly alarmed or psychologically harmed by medical examinations, tests, and treatments. On the contrary, we in Minneapolis have found that torture survivors readily accept appropriate medical care and tolerate medical procedures well. Obviously, certain treatments or procedures (such as dental care in the case of someone who was subjected to dental torture or electrocardiography in the case of someone who was tortured with electric shock) can be psychologically traumatic. But the procedures or treatments can be made tolerable if they are carefully discussed beforehand with a trusted physician or nurse.

Given that many victims of torture come from countries of the world where the psychiatric profession is not well developed and where psychiatrists are rare, torture survivors may be affected by strong cultural taboos about mental illness, mental health care, and psychiatry (Pope and Garcia-Peltoniemi 1991). However, these realities need not be an insurmountable barrier to receiving psychiatric care. The primary care physician can win the trust of the patient and begin to collect a psychiatric history while performing the general medical assessment. For most patients, the primary care physician's role is less threatening and more familiar than that of the psychiatrist. After the medical assessment, most patients accept a referral. The primary care physician can explain that the patient needs a psychiatrist's advice to understand certain physical symptoms and that the psychiatrist has special knowledge of medications to help these symptoms.

Collaboration Between Primary Care and Psychiatry

Although primary care physicians and psychiatrists collaborate closely in the assessment and treatment of patients with complex multisystem medical conditions, they may not be comfortable making diagnoses and prescribing treatments for conditions traditionally within the sphere of the other discipline. When working together on the case of a complex patient such as a victim of torture, physicians in each discipline may be more comfortable compartmentalizing the patient's various problems, categorizing them as either somatic or psychological. In treating torture victims, physicians, including psychiatrists, need to overcome misgivings about visiting unfamiliar professional territory and accept that the patient's medical problems ebb and flow from one discipline to the other, overlapping both. This relationship between primary care physician and psychiatrist is different from the more familiar one in which the psychiatrist is a consultant whose expert opinion is rendered on a one-time basis at the request of the physician treating the case.

Psychiatrists commonly use an approach in which a team of professionals from several disciplines assess and treat a patient. In contrast, primary care physicians tend to see themselves as the sole managers of a particular patient's case, preferring to handle all aspects personally rather than arrange or attend team meetings on treating the patient. When working together to assess and treat victims of torture, primary care physicians and psychiatrists need to clarify management functions and responsibilities.

In conclusion, the relationship between the medical assessment and the subsequent psychiatric care begins when the primary care physician first starts to interact with the torture survivor, and it extends to the point that physical symptoms or medical conditions are resolved or well controlled. The medical assessment is a prelude to the psychiatric care and sets the stage for therapy. In the medical assessment, physical complaints are weighed and placed in context for primary care physician, psychiatrist, and patient. Any operative medical factors that masquerade as psychiatric disorder are identified, and the physical sequelae of torture are objectified. Most important of all, the torture survivor is assured that there are no invisible scars or undetectable damages to fear. The survivor learns that there can be relief from pain, whether that pain be physical or emotional, and that there can be healing and new hope.

References

Basoglu M: Prevention of torture and care of survivors: an integrated approach. JAMA 270:606–611, 1993

Chester B, Holtan N: Working with refugee survivors of torture. Special issue: Cross-cultural medicine—a decade later. West J Med 157:301–304, 1992

Danielsen L, Berger P: Torture located to the skin. Acta Derm Venereol 61:43–46, 1981

Herman JL: Complex PTSD: a syndrome in survivors of prolonged and repeated trauma. J Trauma Stress 5:377–391, 1992

Lifton R: The Nazi Doctors: Medical Killing and the Psychology of Genocide. New York, Basic Books, 1986, p 504

Morris P, Silove D: Cultural influence in psychotherapy with refugee survivors of torture and trauma. Hospital and Community Psychiatry 43:820–824, 1992

Pope K, Garcia-Peltoniemi R: Responding to victims of torture: clinical issues, professional responsibilities, and useful resources. Professional Psychology: Research and Practice 22:269–276, 1991

Skylv G: The physical sequelae of torture, in Torture and Its Consequences: Current Treatment Approaches. Edited by Basoglu M. New York, Cambridge University Press, 1992, pp 38–55

Skylv G: Falange: diagnosis and treatment of late sequelae. Torture 3(1):11–15, 1993

Somnier F, Vesti P, Kastrup M, et al: Psychosocial consequences of torture: current knowledge and evidence, in Torture and Its Consequences: Current Treatment Approaches. Edited by Basoglu M. New York, Cambridge University Press, 1992, pp 56–57

Section IV

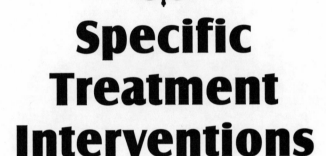

Specific Treatment Interventions

CHAPTER 7

Psychoanalytically Oriented Psychotherapy With Torture Survivors

Sverre Varvin, M.D.
Edvard Hauff, M.D., Ph.D.

If I talked about it, I would feel that it would happen again—
here.

Young refugee from the Middle East

The young woman who made this statement was imprisoned at 20 years of age and went through extreme torture, both physical and psychological. She had been arrested because of minor political activities in high school. The memories associated with the torture were extremely painful, and the thought of talking about them with a therapist seemed unbearable.

In treating victims of torture as well as other victims, we have often encountered situations similar to the one described here. It demonstrates one of the central factors in understanding the phenomenon of trauma. The traumatic experience lives inside the patient like a foreign body, and time seems to be standing still in this area of the personality. It is as though what happened is still continuing. One of the main purposes of therapy is to get the internal clock started so that the trauma can become something in the past. Starting the internal clock will also help the patient secure a future. It is our experience that many patients suffering the consequences of organized violence have difficulty believing that there can be a meaningful future for them. This perspective has multiple determinants, including life in exile with all its attendant anxieties. In this chapter, we concentrate on the trauma experience and its consequences and then offer considerations regarding therapy. If trauma occupies a part of the personality and forces the person to live in the past, how may psychotherapy get things started again?

Our frame of reference is psychodynamic psychotherapy and psychoanalysis, especially object relations theory (Greenberg and Mitchell 1983; Murray Parkes et al. 1991). The therapy we advocate is psychoanalytically oriented therapy. There are special problems connected with the overwhelming experiences of trauma, with cultural differences, and with language differences. We believe that it is possible to help these patients and that the education and experience of Western psychotherapists are good starting points for working with these patients.

Other approaches to the treatment of tortured patients have been described. Cognitive techniques may help patients redefine and reappraise the traumatic experience and develop better cognitive coping techniques (Creamer et al. 1990). A similar effect is reported with a systemic/constructionist approach, in which patient and therapist work to cocreate new meaning related to the trauma, with the result that the patient establishes a new perception of himself or herself (Montgomery 1992).

What distinguishes the psychoanalytical approach is the focus on affect, unconscious representation of traumatic events and their relations to other life events, and aspects of the personality. In addition, the intimate transference relationship allows for working with and possibly repairing damages to the ability for basic trust and internal object relations. Given that cognitive techniques are used within the psychoanalytical approach, one can say that psychoanalytical psychotherapy has a broader focus. Of course, this does not imply that other approaches cannot have beneficial effects and cannot be the treatments of choice for certain patients.

Trauma:
Diagnostic and Psychodynamic Considerations

Trauma was described by Freud (1916–1917/1959) as the overwhelming of the ego with the individual left in a helpless situation. Freud (1920/1959) stressed the incapacity of the ego to deal with impressions from the outside and impulses from within. According to Freud, the traumatic experiences were relived in the mind (e.g., in repetitive dreams), with the purpose of mastering the situation of helplessness. Fairbairn (1954) described trauma in object relations terms. He stressed that the traumatic situation was internalized as an object relation, with the patient partially identifying with the bad object.

Posttraumatic stress disorder (PTSD) has been delineated during the last 10 years, and its symptomatology is well described in DSM-IV (American Psychiatric Association, 1994). The main defense mechanism of this condition appears to be dissociation, and the symptoms of PTSD stem in large part from the failure of this defense mechanism. These symptoms include recurrent dreams in which the traumatic experience is repeated and recurrent intrusions of memories associated with the traumatic situation. Later, what in the traumatic situation was a way of coping becomes a defense mechanism, as the traumatized individual tries to avoid the memories and implications of the traumatic experience.

In a situation with a relatively circumscribed trauma, the object of the treatment (usually psychological debriefing) is to have the patient retell and affectively experience the traumatic situation under safe conditions. This reconstruction must be integrated with the ongoing life situation. This treatment is devised to counteract the persistent dissociation and other deleterious effects of the trauma. It helps the patient to identify the feelings of helplessness and danger that emerged in the traumatic situation. Effects of war traumas and other forms of organized violence may persist for a long time. Multiple traumas can have a cumulative effect (Kahn 1963). This means that the person may not be able to regain strength after a trauma, and this fosters a continuation of dissociation and other defense mechanisms.

The effects of torture and traumas in concentration camps are compounded by the conscious intent to break down and dehumanize the victim (Amati 1987). Torture could be called a kind of therapy in reverse;

its intent is to destroy, rather than build, the personality. We will use the torture experience as the paradigm for the trauma stemming from organized violence.

In the torture situation, the torturer is creating a perverse form of relationship. For the tortured victim, the situation is often experienced as a psychotic-like situation with no possibility of predicting what will happen and no possibility of acting in a way that is in accordance with the tortured person's own moral values and standards and in which there is a constant threat of death. The torturer puts the victim in a dependency situation. The victim experiences an extreme form of helplessness that causes the victim to call on all internal resources, especially the primary internalized caring object, from different phases in infantile development. These childhood objects are imbued with ambivalent qualities. The torturer places himself or herself in a transference-like relationship. Because of the victim's extreme helplessness, the torturer is able to gain access to different aspects of the patient's internal object relations.

It seems that for many patients, the torture situation implies a re-transcription of earlier object relations and what is lost in the torture situation are good childhood memories, those concerning protection by caring parents. Torture evokes problems with attachment, separation, and individuation. The torture situation places a person in a position of extreme helplessness, and in that position he or she will reexperience both the helplessness felt as a child and the strength and caring received as a child. Part of the torturer's purpose is the destruction of the person's internal caring world. Torture creates extreme unreliability; it tends to make both the outer and the inner worlds into chaotic, aggressive spaces. Often, the victim will be forced to act out inner conflicts. In a situation in which a person is forced to give information about family members, early conflicts in relation to these individuals can give rise to extreme guilt feelings. This can take place when the victim has ambivalent feelings toward a parent or sibling.

The external challenges of torture are only a part of the situation. The ego must face aggressive, libidinal impulses. Often there will be situations in which it is almost impossible to integrate what is happening and give it meaning.

According to the Swiss psychoanalyst Amati (1987), torture has three different effects on the personality and the person's life:

- The relation to the body is destroyed. The prisoner has to endure extreme physical pain and stress, such as beating, burning, or electrical stimulation. The victim may be put into water and nearly drowned, or he or she may be starved. Often the prisoner has no options beyond trying to survive.
- The relationships to other persons and to inner objects (inner object relations) are damaged or destroyed. Torture makes ordinary human relations extremely unpredictable and makes them become loaded with aggressive feelings. It compromises meaning.
- The relation to external reality (as defined by space and time) is destroyed by protracted isolation, interruption of sleep, and disruption of the simplest daily routines. These factors compromise the victim's orientation in space and time.

Complex interplays among these three aspects of the torture situation are important to consider when treating these patients.

Dissociation is an important defense mechanism and coping strategy during trauma. Different consequences of dissociation are also present in most patients who have lived through their trauma. There can be depersonalization, derealization, and numbing, among others. Many claim a loss of contact with reality or claim that part of them is, in a way, out of reach. In object relations terms, one can say that the torture creates a split-off part of the personality. The victim has managed to save a normal (or sane) portion of the personality, but the price for this is that a part of the personality has been deformed by the torture experience and resides outside conscious control. For example, one of our patients at the Psychosocial Centre for Refugees, University of Oslo, reported an irresistible desire to bite her husband in social situations. She reported this impulse as ego-alien. It was intense and difficult to resist, exemplifying identification with the aggressor.

We have described how early object relations are activated in the torture situation by the victim's need for comfort and protection. Laub and Auerhahn (1993) reported that a Jewish patient in Auschwitz, during an especially difficult period in the camp, dreamed that her grandmother came, bathed her, and nursed her back to health. When the patient awoke, she felt renewed strength. Such good, early relationships with caring and protective persons are often destroyed by the process of torture and replaced by highly aggressive relationships. All early relationships are marked by a certain ambivalence, and no childhood is without many frustrations. The torturer takes advantage of these realities and can change such protective inner relationships into highly sadomasochistic relationships or near-psychotic relationships. The woman who was quoted at the beginning of this chapter said that to talk about the torture situation would be to relive it during therapy. This means, of course, that many frightening and primitive object relations would be activated in which she could be both the victim of extreme helplessness and the torturer.

The victim of torture tries to keep these experiences out of consciousness. When the trauma is massive, the result may be that parts of the personality are split off and compartmentalized, including highly aggressive tendencies. These isolated or compartmentalized states can come into consciousness during dreams or be experienced in a manner as if in the waking state. This equates to return of the unfavorable or bad object relations.

Needless to say, these states of mind evoke great anxiety. We have described the PTSD-like syndrome linked to different forms of dissociation (Horowitz 1986). There are three additional defensive operations often used when trauma is great and prolonged and the feelings evoked are so violent that the more advanced defense mechanisms are not enough. Primitive anxieties—those concerned with themes of persecution and annihilation—are involved.

Thus, four important defense strategies are employed in the response to the anxiety connected with trauma:

- Dissociation (recurrent nightmares, intrusions)
- Somatization (headaches, pains in different parts of the body, visceral pains)
- Acting out or reduced impulse control (drug or alcohol abuse, aggressiveness, violence)
- Paranoid ideation and possible psychosis

Many manage well as long as they are under the suppressive regime or are in flight. In these situations, it becomes possible to project onto the enemy. On reaching the country of exile, victims are alone with their anxieties (and objects). Somatization seems to be a projection onto the body of very complex conflicts. It can also incorporate elements of the superego that give relief from guilt feelings for having fled. Acting out involves repetition and self-defeating, destructive behavior. Dissociation is a defensive strategy involving the psyche, somatization involves the body, and acting out and psychosis are exteriorizations of mental pain.

Assessment

Several issues must be covered when assessing these patients' suitability for psychotherapy. We find it useful to take as a point of departure the distinction between supportive and expressive therapy. It is common to say that psychotherapies should contain elements of both. As a rule, the less strength present in the patient's ego, the more supportive the therapy must be. The expressive part of the therapy has to do with insight. The coherence and the structure of the ego must be of a certain strength for the split-off parts of the personality to be integrated. The situation when these patients come to treatment is, in our experience, often very insecure and fashioned by the difficulties of the life in exile. Many patients start treatment just after their arrival as refugees. Others come to treatment after several years in a more stable situation. It is important to evaluate the patient's social situation, and there usually must be sufficient safety in the patient's life situation to permit the patient to embark on a systematic therapy. On the other hand, in our experience, many patients have started treatment without this security and have managed to establish a therapeutic relationship. In fact, it seems that for some, therapy was the only way they could establish some security socially.

Severely traumatized people almost always have severe defects in their personality structure and ego-functioning. An initial phase of supportive therapy is often necessary before patients can embark on the more insight-oriented part of therapy.

During assessment of these patients for psychotherapy, consideration must be given to other issues besides motivation and ego-strength. Ideally, patients should be in stable, secure situations. If such is not the case, this problem should, if possible, be dealt with first.

The Therapist

The therapist must ensure that his or her own working conditions are acceptable. Clinical supervision for the therapist should be available. In supervision, the therapist should be able to reflect on his or her own social and cultural position and attitudes related to the patient, in addition to other countertransference issues.

Psychotherapy

Psychotherapy is a meeting between two human beings. It is a very special relationship, often with a strong affective quality. The relatively protected situation, with its regularity and the request to relax and let every thought be expressed permit the patient to concentrate on the internal world. Memories from the past are easier to explore, and mental states connected with these memories can be relived safely. Psychiatric work that was stopped because of sequelae of trauma can be taken up and continued.

There are many realities in such therapeutic relationships. The relationship with the therapist includes a contract of time, duration, and payment. The therapist must be able to give the patient a safe frame for his or her inner voyage. The therapist is a representative for good relationships and the good objects the patient has had in the past. Also, if there have been few such good relationships, or when serious breaks in such relations have occurred, the work to establish this framework of safety becomes more important. In this way, other experiences and mental states can make their way into the therapeutic arena. These can be earlier disappointments with the consequence of mistrust, earlier conflicts in relationships to important others, and the trauma itself, which, as in the above-mentioned woman's experience, foster the maintenance of early negative experiences. In relation to such events, the therapist can also be experienced in a negative way, namely as an unsafe person who can hate, destroy, and take revenge. All these are aspects of transference in psychotherapy.

Among many victims, past traumatic experiences have a very lively character. It can be almost unbearably painful to relive them and work with them in therapy. The woman quoted early in this chapter said that she constantly tried to push the memories of her torture away, but in the dark of evening, when she was tired, she could not resist when they came with renewed strength, making it impossible for her to sleep. For her, as for many others who have experienced torture or catastrophes, this meant a total break with all earlier experiences. It was as though time had stopped, and she reached out for earlier experiences to comfort her, but this was very difficult because too much had been destroyed inside her. The earlier experiences were idealized so that the aggressive parts could be kept away; but she could not manage this for longer periods. She had to be affirmed constantly by the therapist or by telephone calls to her family in her home country.

There are three important aspects to be considered when planning and doing therapy.

- First of all, consideration must be given to the patient's somatic health. It is important to have the cooperation of a general practitioner who can treat or address the somatic illnesses that may occur. In this type of therapy, one must look after the bodily welfare of the patient in a concrete way, seeing that he or she is not uncomfortable in the situation. Psychosomatic illness, conversion symptoms, and somatization are important aspects of the symptomatology. These are expressions of internal psychic conflicts. The following case example illustrates this point.

A South American woman in exile sought therapy at the Psychosocial Centre for Refugees, University of Oslo, several years after she had been severely tortured. One of her physical complaints was frequent and incapacitating migraine attacks. When this symptom was explored, it turned out that the attacks often occurred at a certain time during the night and that they woke her. She denied that she ever remembered any dreams. The patient and the therapist adopted a working hypothesis that the attacks were related to her dream experiences and, more specifically, that dreams about the torture might precipitate them. When a sufficient working alliance had been formed, the patient started to report dreams in the sessions. They frequently contained material related to her incarceration, the torture, and her subsequent traumatic losses. The material usually appeared in a symbolic form, and the content was thus not a mere repetition of the traumatic events. After she began reporting her dreams, her migraine attacks subsided and finally disappeared.

- With regard to the patient's relation to time and space, it is very important to create a safe and secure setting for the therapy with such things as regular meetings and fixed length of appointments. Even if the patient, especially in the beginning of therapy, can meet only irregularly, it is important to maintain fixed appointments. One patient, even after prolonged therapy with regular hours, could not believe that the therapist continued to meet with him after the patient skipped a single session.
- It is also important to bear in mind the effects on the patient of not being able to perform usual habits and rituals and being denied routine sleep during time in captivity. The patient may have developed a psychotic-like anxiety, which also makes it difficult for the patient, when released from prison, to reestablish important aspects of normal everyday life (Werbart and Lindbom-Jacobson 1993).

With a therapy structured according to object relations theory, it is important to address transference phenomena as they emerge in therapy. When split-off parts come into the relationship, it is important to ensure that this occurs under secure conditions.

Although systematic studies are lacking, clinical experiences indicate that certain therapeutic attitudes and interventions are particularly helpful in facilitating the therapeutic process. In the initial phase, these include providing information to the patient about the purpose and method of psychotherapy, which must be adjusted to the patient's sociocultural background. The main focus is to establish a sufficient working alliance; usually a trusting relationship will develop very slowly. This means that it is important to work on the relationship and the therapeutic setting to make the patient feel safe. Material directly and indirectly related to torture or other experiences of organized violence is presented throughout the therapy in a variety of forms. The therapist must stress that it will be explained indirectly both in relation to the therapist and in reaction to other important persons in the patient's life.

Shame and guilt feelings are very important. The former is a painful feeling, but for severely tortured patients it can be a sign of a more human way of relating to other people (Sas 1992). Aggressive fantasies are often directed toward the therapist and others and can be in the form of constant devaluation or more prolonged negative therapeutic reactions. The possibilities for exploring and interpreting internalized conflicts are related to the patient's personality development and the relationship of the conflicts to his or her reaction to the trauma. Explorations in this area seem to be better in the middle and later phases of therapy, after a solid and stable relationship has developed. A case example of a patient who felt guilt and exhibited aggressive behavior toward his therapist follows.

An exiled teacher from a country in the Middle East had been sexually abused in adolescence and was bitter and angry with his father, whom he felt had not protected him sufficiently during that period of his life. Later he was arrested for political reasons and was tortured in prison. During therapy, he brought material related to both these traumatic periods. This material was also explored in relation to earlier (oedipal) conflicts and to his experiences in exile. But he often felt overwhelmed by anger, and the interventions were often supportive and focused on his abilities to cope with the adversities of exile.

He also suffered from posttraumatic dissociative symptoms that impaired his work performance, and at one stage he requested a medical certificate from the psychiatrist concerning this. When the therapist did not comply, the patient got very angry, devalued the whole therapy, and stated that he would leave therapy. The therapist said that he would honor their next appointment, and he advised the patient to do the same. When the patient returned, he described the guilt he had felt immediately after the last session, and he compared this reaction to feelings he had toward his father. He was now able to continue to explore these feelings, also in the context of the transference to the therapist. In addition, they discussed the realities of the therapeutic contract and its possible shortcomings.

Issues related to the patient's exile situation, minority position, and acculturation are likely to be expressed and should be addressed both in relation to the real-life situations and in association with fantasies and transference.

What we usually call the supportive aspect of psychotherapy will be very significant with these patients. Especially in the beginning phase of therapy, the supportive elements must prevail. One should never forget that these patients are always vulnerable to rejection, maltreatment, and disrespect.

It is our experience that psychopharmacological treatment can go hand in hand with psychotherapy. When the therapist is a physician, there are not many problems with concurrently administrating psychopharmacological treatment. During periods of the therapy when the patient has great anxiety of a delusional kind (e.g., is afraid of being attacked or spied on), small doses of antipsychotic medicine can help; likewise, if the patient has clear depressive episodes, antidepressants can be helpful. As an alternative, referral may be arranged with another doctor who provides psychopharmacological treatment.

There is always a question of whether one should embark on long-term therapy or restrict treatment to a focal therapy of limited length. Most of the literature on therapy with traumatized patients points to the trauma as the focus of interest. However, we have found that it is very important to pay attention to the patient's earlier experiences, because what is lost during torture are often the good relationships that the patient had earlier with important others. These relationships can help the patient restore his or her faith and belief in self and also serve as a buffer against the horrible, traumatic experiences that can dominate. When formulating a focus for a more limited therapy, one must bear in mind therefore that an exclusive focus on the trauma may be too great a burden to the patient.

Although the structure and content of the therapy may vary, the reconnection with good objects and self-representations probably is the most important feature of psychotherapy with patients who have survived torture and other forms of organized violence (Herman 1992). These relationships also need nurturing and development during therapy. Such a process is obviously demanding both for the patient and for the therapist. But it is likely to be deeply meaningful for both of them and a chance for the patient to move from the position of powerless victim to that of active survivor.

References

Amati S: Some thoughts on torture. Free Associations 8:94–114, 1987
American Psychiatric Association: Diagnostic and Statistical Manual of Mental Disorders, 4th Edition. Washington, DC, American Psychiatric Association, 1994

Creamer M, Burgess P, Pattison P: Cognitive processing in post-traumatic reactions: some preliminary findings. Psychol Med 20:579–604, 1990

Fairbairn WRD: An Object-Relations Theory of the Personality. New York, Basic Books, 1954

Freud S: Five lectures in Psychoanalysis and other works (1916–1917), in Standard Edition of the Complete Psychological Works of Sigmund Freud, Vol 11. Translated and edited by Strachey J. London, Hogarth Press, 1959, p 284

Freud S: Totem and taboo and other works (1916–1917), in Standard Edition of the Complete Psychological Works of Sigmund Freud, Vol 13. Translated and edited by Strachey J. London, Hogarth Press, 1959, pp 1–69

Greenberg JR, Mitchell SA: Object Relations in Psychoanalytic Theory. Cambridge, MA, Harvard University Press, 1983

Herman JL: Trauma and Recovery: The Aftermath of Violence—From Domestic Abuse to Political Terror. New York, Basic Books, 1992

Horowitz MD: Stress Response Syndromes, 2nd Edition. Northvale, NJ, Jason Aronson, 1986

Kahn MMR: The concept of cumulative trauma, in The British School of Psychoanalysis: The Independent Tradition. Edited by Kohon G. London, Free Association Books, 1963

Laub D, Auerhahn NC: Knowing and not knowing massive psychic trauma: forms of traumatic memory. Int J Psychoanal 74:287–302, 1993

Montgomery E: Co-creation of meaning in therapy with torture survivors: a systemic/constructionist view. Human Systems: The Journal of Systemic Consultation and Management 3:27–33, 1992

Murray Parkes C, Stevenson-Hinde J, Marris P: Attachment Across the Life Cycle. London, Tavistock/Routledge, 1991

Sas SA: Ambiguity as the route to shame. Int J Psychoanal 73:329–341, 1992

Werbart A, Lindbom-Jacobson M: The "living dead"—survivors of torture and psychosis. Psychoanalytic Psychotherapy 7:163–179, 1993

CHAPTER 8

Behavioral and Cognitive Treatment of Survivors of Torture

Metin Başoğlu, M.D., Ph.D.

In the last decade, there has been a surge of interest in the problems of survivors of torture. Numerous care and rehabilitation centers for survivors have been set up in various parts of the world. The rehabilitation models used by these centers are often determined by the sociopolitical circumstances of the country in which the centers are based and by the political and professional orientation of the staff (van Willigen 1992).

Psychodynamic psychotherapy appears to be a widely used method for treating torture survivors. Alternative methods include various other forms of individual and group psychotherapy. A three-phase form of psychotherapy described by Somnier and Genefke (1986) involves cognitive restructuring, emotional reconstruction of trauma, and reestablishment of reality. This approach is based on the principle that a systematic working through or emotional reconstruction of the traumatic events results in a reintegration of the traumatic experience and subsequent alleviation of symptoms. In the "testimony" method (Agger and Jensen 1990; Cienfuegos and Monelli 1983), the survivor provides a detailed account of the torture experience in the form of a written testimony.

So far, there is little evidence regarding the effectiveness of a particular treatment approach for survivors of torture (Basoglu and Marks 1988). There are no controlled studies of the efficacy of currently available treatment methods. Most descriptions of psychological treatments are not adequately detailed. Many appear to consist of various therapeutic elements and lack a theoretical basis. Outcome evaluations are not based on systematic measurement of problem areas with adequate follow-up. It is therefore difficult to draw conclusions on the efficacy of these treatments.

In this chapter, I review the evidence for the efficacy of behavioral and cognitive treatment in posttraumatic stress disorder (PTSD), outline the basic principles of treatment for survivors of torture, and present a case example to illustrate the approach. A more detailed description of the treatment techniques and a discussion of their theoretical rationale have been reported elsewhere (Basoglu 1992). (See also Basoglu and Mineka [1992] for a learning theory account of traumatic stress responses in survivors of torture.) Also presented in this chapter is a discussion of the elements that behavioral treatment and other widely used psychotherapies in the field have in common. The search for common elements between various psychotherapies based on different theoretical formulations is important because the differences between them may be more apparent than real. Identification of the therapeutic ingredients shared by various treatment approaches could further the understanding of the underlying mechanisms of traumatic stress responses and help improve our treatment techniques.

Behavioral and Cognitive Treatment of Posttraumatic Stress Disorder

Behavior therapy is based on the principle that prolonged imaginal or live exposure to an anxiety-evoking situation reduces anxiety. Evidence for the efficacy of exposure-based treatments in PTSD was initially based on single case studies, mainly of Vietnam combat veterans (Black and Keane 1982; Fairbank and Keane 1982; Fairbank et al. 1981, 1983; Keane and Kaloupek 1982). Controlled studies demonstrated the efficacy of behavioral treatments in combat-related PTSD. In a randomized controlled trial

(Cooper and Clum 1989), only flooding achieved significant improvement; this improvement was maintained at 3-month follow-up. In a second study (Keane et al. 1989), results of implosive therapy were superior to those of no therapy (in a wait-list control group) immediately after treatment and at 6-month follow-up. In a third study (Boudewyns and Hyer 1990), imaginal flooding achieved greater improvement than counseling. Imaginal exposure was also found effective in four patients with PTSD who had suffered other types of traumas (Richards and Rose 1991). Clearly, behavioral treatments are promising in the treatment of stress responses induced by a variety of traumatic events.

These treatments, however, appear to have a differential effect on PTSD symptoms. Positive symptoms such as intrusive recollections, nightmares, reexperiencing of the trauma, sleep disturbance, irritability, and startle response seem to be more responsive to exposure-based treatments than negative symptoms such as emotional numbing and estrangement (Keane 1989). A stress management approach that includes relaxation training, cognitive restructuring, and problem-solving skills training may be needed to improve the residual symptoms (Keane et al. 1985).

The effectiveness of cognitive therapy in PTSD has not yet been investigated (Blake et al. 1990). Although some treatment approaches for survivors of torture involve cognitive interventions (Somnier and Genefke 1986; Vesti and Kastrup 1992), their efficacy in the treatment of torture-induced PTSD remains to be demonstrated. However, cognitive therapy may be valuable for treating the depression that is so often part of the clinical picture in torture survivors and for treating the negative symptoms (e.g., guilt, estrangement, loss of meaning, emotional numbing) that may not have responded to exposure treatment (Basoglu 1992).

Behavioral Treatment for Torture Survivors

Preparation for treatment. Assessment of suitability and motivation for treatment is crucial because treatment success depends largely on the survivor's compliance with and active participation in treatment. A full understanding of the treatment rationale and a willingness to go through the initial distressing phase of treatment are essential. Reeducation of the survivor regarding the nature of the symptoms and their impact on social functioning can help not only to enhance motivation for treatment but also to alleviate some of the symptoms. Some survivors may not be aware of the connection between the traumatic experience and psychological or somatic symptoms. Reeducation, then, helps the survivor understand how his or her complaints, particularly the somatic symptoms, relate to the torture experience. Once the survivor has such an understanding, he or she is ready for a discussion of treatment method and aims.

The survivor also needs to understand fully that the reason for confronting anxiety-evoking situations and memories is to allow anxiety and other painful emotions to subside. Avoidance of reminders of past trauma only serves to sustain the symptoms. Provided that exposure to anxiety cues is of sufficient duration, the anxiety evoked by these situations does not last forever and eventually subsides. This understanding is crucial because much of the treatment outside therapy sessions consists of homework sessions involving self-initiated exposure.

The critical step in preparation for treatment is a careful behavioral analysis of the most distressing and disabling problem areas. These are often the positive symptoms of PTSD, such as intrusive recollections of the trauma, fear and avoidance of trauma-related cues, generalized anxiety and/or panic, startle reactions, irritability, outbursts of anger and hostility, and nightmares. The internal and external cues that trigger the distressing symptoms are identified, and the links between symptoms and socially disordered behavior are clarified. This process often provides valuable information about the most traumatic aspects of the survivor's past experience and how they relate to present problems. Once the problem areas are identified, they are set as the targets of treatment. Care needs to be taken to set treatment targets of which the patient approves, because much will depend on the patient's own initiative and active participation in the treatment.

Treatment sessions.   The treatment consists mainly of two components: implosive therapy, or flooding, and in vivo exposure.

Implosive therapy involves an imaginal reconstruction of traumatic events in an emotionally supportive therapy context. The patient is asked to imagine the traumatic situations and retain the trauma-related imagery in mind until anxiety diminishes. The therapist helps sustain the state of mental arousal by presenting two types of cues: 1) trauma-specific stimuli that involve imagery related to the forms of torture used, the physical and psychological pain experienced, and other aspects of the torture situation, such as sounds, sights, smells, and tactile sensations; and 2) conditioned stimuli relating to the individual's cognitive and emotional responses to torture, such as fear, guilt, self-blame, humiliation, shame, and loss of control. The latter are particularly important because torture is often deliberately designed to produce such emotions.

Sessions, usually lasting 1½ to 2 hours, initially take place two or three times a week. The total number of sessions may vary according to the needs of the individual but is usually between 10 and 20. All traumatic aspects of the torture experience should be covered before termination of treatment so that antitherapeutic effects arising from incomplete or partial exposure to trauma cues are avoided. When feasible, sessions may be audiotaped for use in homework exercises between sessions. Homework consists of listening to the taped material over and over until it no longer evokes intense anxiety. This technique has also been found helpful in PTSD related to other types of trauma (Richards and Rose 1991).

In vivo exposure is often useful in treating fear and avoidance of various situations—a problem that may be extremely distressing and socially incapacitating. Torture survivors with PTSD often show anxiety and avoidance responses to a variety of situations that resemble the torture experience (Bøjholm and Vesti 1992). Electrical torture, for instance, may lead to avoidance of electric appliances or medical procedures such as electroencephalography or electrocardiography. Sexually tortured survivors may avoid gynecological examinations or sexual relationships. Solitary confinement may result in a fear of closed spaces. Authority figures, people in uniform, police stations, government offices, or hospitals may evoke panic and avoidance. Sometimes agoraphobia-like conditions may occur, with survivors becoming housebound.

In vivo exposure consists of incremental exposure to anxiety-evoking situations until anxiety disappears. During the first few sessions, the therapist may need to accompany the survivor into avoided situations to provide encouragement and support. The frequency at which the patient is exposed to avoided situations may be increased according to his or her needs. Some patients may require a more gradual pace of exposure than others to keep anxiety within tolerable limits during each task.

Once the patient is ready to undertake further exposure tasks without therapist assistance, the treatment continues as self-exposure with regular evaluation of progress and setting of new targets. Throughout treatment, the survivor is given strong emotional support, encouragement, and verbal praise for any progress made. Exposure homework is crucial for reinforcing any improvement achieved during the treatment sessions. The patient is thus asked to continue doing homework between sessions. The details concerning each exposure task are recorded in a homework diary so that the therapist can monitor progress at the next session.

Cognitive Treatment for Torture Survivors

As noted earlier, behavioral treatment may leave negative symptoms of PTSD unresolved or only partially resolved in some trauma survivors (Keane 1989; Keane et al. 1992). (These symptoms include guilt, low self-esteem, self-blame, feelings of estrangement, and emotional numbing.) However, anxiety extinction during implosive therapy is often accompanied or followed by cognitive change without any active cognitive intervention (Basoglu 1992). Nevertheless, cognitive therapy may be useful in dealing with problems that persist after behavioral treatment.

Torture is often designed to remove total control and induce feelings of helplessness in the individual. The role of uncontrollable stressors in producing feelings of helplessness in survivors of torture has been reviewed in detail elsewhere (Basoglu and Mineka 1992). Individuals experience varying degrees of loss of control during torture, and this may explain why some survivors have persistent feelings of helplessness and others do not.

Attributional theory (Abramson et al. 1978), which distinguishes between internal and external, global and specific, and stable and unstable attributions, also appears to be useful in explaining varying individual responses to uncontrollable stress during torture. Survivors who attribute the cause of uncontrollable traumatic events to themselves (internal attribution), generalize them across situations (global attribution), and perceive them to be chronic (stable attribution) seem to be more likely to have more severe problems. Survivors who believe that they have failed to cope with torture or that they behaved in an undignified manner to prevent further torture may see their failure as a sign of weakness in their character rather than as a normal human response to extreme trauma. Such beliefs may generate considerable guilt, shame, self-blame, and social withdrawal.

Cognitive intervention in such cases involves encouraging survivors to think that their behavior under torture was a normal, human response necessary for survival; that torture is designed to induce total loss of control and helplessness, which may explain why they behaved the way they did; that they may have been deliberately forced to make impossible choices; that most individuals experience helplessness under extreme stress and that this is not necessarily a sign of weakness in one's character. Behaviors regarded as mistakes are identified, and self-statements associating blame with one's character (e.g., "I am weak and untrustworthy") are replaced by self-statements that attribute mistakes to one's behavior (e.g., "I made a mistake; it was my carelessness").

The following statements may also be useful in shifting the focus of the blame: 1) "Individuals cannot be held entirely responsible for involuntary acts committed under extreme coercion"; 2) "It is the torturers who should be blamed for having committed such atrocities. I should be able to speak out freely about my experience because the degrading treatment I went through degrades only the torturers"; and 3) "Torture is deliberately designed to undermine one's self-respect and dignity. Therefore, blaming myself for what happened is an admission of the torturers' victory."

Certain PTSD symptoms, such as suspiciousness, generalized mistrust of others, estrangement, a feeling of loss of meaning in life, and emotional numbing, may be related in part to violations of basic assumptions about other human beings and the world in general. That the world is just (the *just-world hypothesis* [Staub 1990]) and that it is a safe place in which to live are common basic assumptions. Violations of basic concepts of safety are thought to be associated with PTSD (Foa et al. 1989).

Two approaches may be taken in dealing with these psychological problems. In some cases, it may be useful to help the survivor recover original assumptions about the world and original perceptions of safety. Most rehabilitation programs and psychotherapies appear to achieve this aim, either directly or indirectly, by creating a secure and stable therapy environment in which the survivor can begin to learn to trust others and to regain his or her sense of security. For example, through physical contact with the therapist during physiotherapy sessions, he or she can learn to trust physical closeness with others and understand that not all physical contact signals danger. Establishing a trusting relationship with the therapist may also help restore basic trust in others.

An alternate approach might be to help the survivor to come to terms with living without any assumptions about the world. The world is neither a totally safe or just place nor a totally unsafe or unjust place, and human beings are neither completely trustworthy nor completely untrustworthy. To take either position is to have a distorted view of reality. It might help to think in terms of probabilities in explaining why things happen to people. For instance, in dealing with the question "Why did this happen to me?" one might think, "If disasters are happening in the world, they have to happen to some people, and there is no reason to assume they will not happen to me." One can exert some control over undesirable events, but the probability of their occurrence can never be entirely eliminated. Safety is thus a transient state of probabilities, only sometimes in favor of one's well-being. Life is a series of actions involving risk, and one cannot constantly dwell on the dangers involved at each step.

The question of whether human beings deserve one's trust can be dealt with in a similar fashion. Given the right circumstances, human beings are capable of inflicting great pain on each other, although some are perhaps more prone to do this than others. The belief that human beings are essentially good, although this belief may generally serve a useful purpose, is an illusion. A discussion along these lines may help the survivor to achieve a more realistic perception of the world, one not involving recourse to dichotomies of good and evil, trustworthy and untrustworthy, and safe and unsafe. This approach is based on the understanding that the highly traumatic experience of torture can transform into a useful learning experience or result in a positive outcome through helping the survivor shed illusory perceptions of the world and acquire a more realistic outlook.

Generalized suspiciousness and mistrust of others observed in some survivors seem to stem from an overestimation of the probability of physical or psychological threat in the environment. Cognitive interventions aimed at correcting the distortions in probability estimation may be useful in treating such symptoms. Successful exposure to situations in which the estimated probability of danger is unrealistically high often leads to concomitant reduction in threat expectancy without any cognitive intervention. One of my patients made a point of going into police stations with an excuse and spending time chatting with the officers. The friendly chat enabled him to overcome his generalized fear of authority by helping him to think that the presence of police did not always signal danger. He reported that after this discovery, there was a marked reduction in his mistrust of authority and in the overall estimation of danger in his environment.

Certain cognitive techniques may be useful in dealing with symptoms such as irritability, outbursts of anger and aggressiveness, and other behavioral problems that undermine social adaptation (Keane et al. 1992). These involve helping the patient to identify the negative self-statements that trigger maladaptive behavior and replace them with positive self-statements. Anxiety management strategies could also be beneficial with regard to these problems.

Behavioral and Cognitive Treatment of PTSD Symptoms in a Survivor of Torture: A Case Report

The following describes the case of a patient who was treated first with behavior therapy and then with cognitive therapy.

A 25-year-old African man who was involved in political unrest in his country was arrested by security forces, detained for 1 day, and tortured. He subsequently fled his country and applied for political asylum in England in 1989. After settling in England, he enrolled in a polytechnic school to continue his higher education. In mid-1989, he developed a psychotic illness, presenting as persecutory delusions and aggressive and violent behavior. He was admitted to a psychiatric hospital.

On psychiatric examination, he was found to have abnormal perceptions, including perceptions of people coming to get him and of being followed by people whom he could not always see but whose presence he could feel. He reported voices shouting obscenities in his ear and experienced thought blocking, somatic passivity, and thought broadcasting. Results of laboratory testing and techniques including Venereal Disease Research Laboratory testing, electroencephalography, and computed tomography (CT) were unremarkable. He was diagnosed as having a paranoid psychosis (unspecified), and haloperidol therapy was started.

The patient's psychotic symptoms resolved within 2 months, after which time he was referred to me for treatment of PTSD symptoms. He had trauma-related complaints whose onset predated the psychotic episode. These complaints included nightmares about his torture that made him wake up in terror, distress on being reminded of the trauma, avoidance of activities that made him remember past events (e.g., watching news on TV, reading newspapers), unwillingness to talk about painful memories, social withdrawal, and inability to give a meaning to his traumatic experience.

First, a behavioral approach was used to deal with the positive symptoms of PTSD. He was told that talking about the trauma and prolonged exposure to situations that brought back memories of torture might be painful in the beginning but would eventually reduce his distress. He fully understood the treatment rationale and expressed satisfactory motivation for treatment.

Imaginal exposure was initially conducted with considerable care and in a limited and graduated fashion because of his recent psychotic episode. Emotional arousal during the first session, however, was not intense enough to cause concern. The trauma material was covered in detail in three sessions, with considerable reduction in associated distress. He was able to talk about his torture experience freely. As his homework, he was asked to read all newspapers in the ward and cut clippings of news about human rights abuses and file them. In the next session, he would read these pieces of news again and discuss them with the therapist.

He quickly became habituated to the distress involved in this task, but news about African countries still continued to cause some discomfort because they closely resembled the events in his home country. He was then asked to write to Amnesty International and request the latest report on the political events in his country. When he received the report, his task was to read through the 40-page document daily until there was significant reduction in his distress. He was asked to rate within-session peak anxiety at the end of each homework session, using a visual analog scale that ranged from *no distress at all* to *extreme distress.*

Daily ratings were averaged to obtain a weekly rating of anxiety level over a 6-week period. Despite considerable reduction in task-related anxiety over 6 weeks, the patient's anxiety did not fall to a zero level. This is understandable given that anxiety cues in traumatic stress response syndromes, unlike other anxiety disorders, often concern events or situations that would be expected to evoke emotional responses in psychiatrically healthy individuals. The reduction in task-related distress was of sufficient magnitude, however, to achieve a clinically significant improvement in the patient's condition.

Reduction in general anxiety also led to a reduction in the number of nightmares, although they did not disappear completely. The patient was then given the additional task of recording in detail in his diary every nightmare he had experienced. The nightmares had a recurrent theme and related to the original trauma (that of being chased, caught, and tortured by government soldiers). He would then go through the details of the nightmare several times during the day until he no longer felt distressed.

At the end of behavioral treatment, the patient was able to discuss his traumatic experiences with other patients and staff without difficulty and was able to read newspapers, watch TV, and engage in any other activity that reminded him of his past trauma. By this time his nightmares had disappeared completely. The change in his behavior was also noted by the ward staff. At this stage, cognitive therapy was started to aid him in understanding the meaning of his traumatic experience. He was helped gradually to become aware of the fact that what happened to him in his country was a part of the gross human rights violations throughout the world that are endured by millions of people and that he was not unique in his experience. He was given a reading list of works, including Amnesty International publications, on human rights abuses in various countries. These interventions helped him to see his torture experience in the broader perspective of human rights violations in the world and to depersonalize the traumatic experience.

The whole treatment process required seven sessions over a period of 3 months. After treatment, he stopped taking medication and was discharged from the hospital. At 3-month follow-up, he was free of any psychotic or posttraumatic stress symptoms.

A number of conclusions can be drawn from the results seen in this case:

- In traumatized individuals, PTSD symptoms may persist after recovery from a psychotic illness and may need further treatment.
- Behavioral approaches shown to be effective in PTSD may also be useful in treating survivors of torture, as demonstrated by other case studies of behavioral treatment in torture survivors (Basoglu and Aker 1996; Yüksel 1989). Improvement in PTSD symptoms in this patient led to an

improved social functioning, as observed by the ward staff.

- Behavioral treatment can be applied to traumatized individuals who have a recent history of psychotic illness, provided that the rate of exposure is conducted at a slower pace than usual so that anxiety is kept within tolerable limits. Concomitant neuroleptic treatment may also help keep anxiety under control.

- Learning that takes place under the effect of medication (haloperidol in the case example) may be transferred to a nondrug state; in the case example, improvement was maintained during drug-free follow-up.

- The improvement in positive symptoms may be achieved by a behavioral approach without any active cognitive intervention. In the case example, cognitive therapy was started toward the end of behavior therapy, after the positive symptoms had resolved.

- Finally, significant improvement in PTSD symptoms can be achieved in a relatively brief time.

Parallels Between Various Psychotherapies

Most psychotherapy methods used in treating trauma survivors, including psychodynamic psychotherapy, have a common goal: the integration of the traumatic experience through emotional reconstruction or a therapeutic reliving of the trauma (Agger 1989; Agger and Jensen 1990; Allodi 1986; Blackburn et al. 1984; Brende 1981; Brende and McCann 1984; Cienfuegos and Monelli 1983; Crump 1984; Garcia-Peltoniemi and Jaranson 1989; Horowitz 1973, 1974; Horowitz et al. 1984; Ortmann et al. 1987; Roth et al. 1987; Somnier and Genefke 1986; Vesti and Kastrup 1992). Such integration is achieved by getting the survivor to talk about the traumatic experience. This goal also applies to behavioral procedures involving imaginal exposure to the trauma. It is possible, therefore, that the therapeutic effect of all these methods is achieved through imaginal exposure to trauma memories and consequent extinction of anxiety. Cognitive change necessary for the integration of the traumatic experience may either accompany or follow the process of extinction.

A closer look at some of the methods used in treating torture survivors reveals striking similarities to the behavioral approach. The testimony method (Agger and Jensen 1990; Cienfuegos and Monelli 1983) developed in Chile in the 1970s is a treatment involving 3 to 10 sessions of tape-recording of the details of detention, torture, and other political suffering, with emphasis on particularly significant traumatic events. In the study described by Cienfuegos and Monelli (1983), the audiotape was then transcribed as a 15- to 120-page text and reviewed with the survivors for editing. Among the 39 tortured ex-prisoners and other persons who suffered nontorture trauma, the best results were achieved with persons whose traumas concerned torture (12 of 15 such individuals improved). The audiotaping, transcription, review, and editing of a 15- to 120-page text clearly involves many hours of imaginal exposure to the traumatic experience.

Similarities to the behavioral approach can be found in the descriptions of rehabilitation programs for torture survivors as well (e.g., Bøjholm and Vesti 1992). These programs involve a fair amount of medical investigation, ranging from physical examinations, blood tests, electroencephalography, and electrocardiography to more extensive procedures such as gastroscopy, proctoscopy, dental treatment, and surgery. Physiotherapy is an integral part of the treatment and takes place in a physical setting that may involve closed spaces, application of various instruments to the body, water, nakedness, doctors, and authority figures. These procedures and situations, through their apparent similarity to the torture situation, may serve as conditioned-fear stimuli and thus provide ample opportunity for exposure and habituation to occur. Survivors are said to show intense anxiety and have emotional reactions to these procedures.

What are the critical psychotherapeutic ingredients in cognitive-behavioral treatment, the testimony method, or rehabilitation programs for torture survivors: cognitive change or anxiety extinction through exposure or both? It is possible that cognitive intervention, even when no overt behavioral exposure is involved, has an effect through imaginal exposure. Controlled studies in anxiety disorders comparing cognitive-behavioral treatment with exposure alone have found no significant differences in outcome (Emmelkamp and Mersch 1982; Emmelkamp et al. 1978, 1985; Mavissakalian et al. 1983; Williams and Rappoport 1983). Similarly, there is as yet no evidence for the efficacy of cognitive therapy in PTSD (Blake et al. 1990). On the other hand, the fact that significant improvement can be achieved through exposure alone in PTSD, as well as in other anxiety disorders, suggests an important role for exposure. Exposure may be the ingredient that initiates emotional processing (Rachman 1980) and cognitive change (Foa and Kozak 1986). The cognitive therapist's role may be to remove the barriers (e.g., cognitive avoidance, absence of short-term habituation, depression, overvalued ideation) to optimal emotional processing (Foa and Kozak 1986).

Conclusion

Behavior therapy is a promising treatment for PTSD in general, and there is preliminary evidence for its usefulness in treating torture-related psychological problems. In addition, behavioral treatment has some distinct advantages that deserve attention here. First, it is a brief form of psychotherapy, which makes it particularly suitable for clinical practice in parts of the world where torture is widespread, rehabilitation centers are nonexistent, and the individual practitioner, faced with many trauma survivors in need, must act on his or her own. Long-term psychotherapies may not be feasible; in South Africa, for example, many survivors are unable to maintain contact with mental health professionals after the first interview (Dowdall 1992).

Second, knowledge of behavioral techniques can be easily disseminated to parts of the world where action is urgently needed. Training in behavioral psychology is relatively easy and is less time consuming than training in most other methods. Anyone can be trained in behavioral methods—social workers, nurses, psychiatrists, psychologists, and other health professionals. Given the extent and urgency of the problem, speed of delivery of services is an important consideration. In countries where there are thousands of survivors of organized violence and torture, the best course of action is to train local mental health professionals, volunteer groups, and even the survivors themselves in behavioral techniques. These techniques can also be used effectively in a group context, which would further speed up the delivery of services. In addition, behavioral treatment can be easily packaged in the form of self-help manuals or brochures, and, where feasible, its principles can be disseminated to the public through radio, TV, and other mass media.

The goal-oriented approach of behavior therapy has led some to believe that it is a limited or superficial form of treatment. Although no single treatment is a panacea for the wide range of psychological and social problems associated with organized violence and torture, such a belief reflects a misconception. As noted earlier, behavioral treatment focuses on the most important and disabling problem areas in the individual's life. The improvement achieved by behavioral treatment in physiological, behavioral, and cognitive problem areas often generalizes to social, family, marital, and work problems and improves quality of life. Furthermore, as follow-up studies of anxiety disorders have shown, these effects are lasting ones (Foa and Kozak 1986; Foa et al. 1989). Finally, the emphasis of the behavioral approach on careful assessment allows testing of hypotheses concerning its efficacy, a fundamental requirement for any scientific endeavor.

References

Abramson LY, Seligman MEP, Teasdale SJ: Learned helplessness in humans: critique and reformulation. J Abnorm Psychol 87:49–94, 1978

Agger I: Sexual torture of political prisoners: an overview. J Trauma Stress 2:305–318, 1989

Agger I, Jensen SB: Testimony as ritual and evidence in psychotherapy for political refugees. J Trauma Stress 3:115–130, 1990

Allodi F: Psychotherapy of posttraumatic stress disorders: a multicultural model. Abstract of paper presented at the Workshop on Mass Violence and Posttraumatic Stress Disorders, Rockville, MD, April 14–15, 1986

Basoglu M: Behavioral and cognitive treatment of PTSD in torture survivors, in Torture and Its Consequences: Current Treatment Approaches. Edited by Basoglu M. New York, Cambridge University Press, 1992, pp 402–429

Basoglu M, Aker T: Cognitive-behavioural treatment of torture survivors: a case study. Torture 6:61–65, 1996

Basoglu M, Marks IM: Torture. BMJ 297:1423–1424, 1988

Basoglu M, Mineka S: The role of uncontrollability and unpredictability of stress in the development of posttorture stress symptoms, in Torture and Its Consequences: Current Treatment Approaches. Edited by Basoglu M. New York, Cambridge University Press, 1992, pp 182–225

Black JL, Keane TM: Implosive therapy in the treatment of combat related fears in a World War II veteran. J Behav Ther Exp Psychiatry 13:163–165, 1982

Blackburn AB, O'Connell WE, Richman BW: PTSD, the Vietnam veteran and Adlerian natural high therapy. Individual psychology. Journal of Individual Psychology 40:317–332, 1984

Blake DD, Albano AM, Keane TM: Trends in trauma: psychology abstracts 1970 to 1990. Abstract of paper presented at the 6th annual meeting of the Society for Traumatic Stress Studies, New Orleans, LA, October 28–31, 1990

Bøjholm S, Vesti P: Multidisciplinary approach in the treatment of torture survivors, in Torture and Its Consequences: Current Treatment Approaches. Edited by Basoglu M. New York, Cambridge University Press, 1992, pp 299–309

Boudewyns PA, Hyer L: Physiological response in combat veterans and preliminary treatment in Vietnam PTSD patients treated with direct therapeutic exposure. Behav Res Ther 21:63–87, 1990

Brende JO: Combined individual and group therapy for Vietnam veterans. International Journal of Psychotherapy 31:367–378, 1981

Brende JO, McCann IL: Regressive experiences in Vietnam veterans: their relationship to war, posttraumatic symptoms and recovery. Journal of Contemporary Psychotherapy 14:57–75, 1984

Cienfuegos AJ, Monelli C: The testimony of political repression as a therapeutic instrument. Am J Orthopsychiatry 53:43–51, 1983

Cooper NA, Clum GA: Imaginal flooding as a supplementary treatment for PTSD in combat veterans: a controlled study. Behav Res Ther 20:381–391, 1989

Crump LE: Gestalt therapy in the treatment of Vietnam veterans experiencing PTSD symptomatology. Journal of Contemporary Psychotherapy 14:90–98, 1984

Dowdall T: Torture and the helping professions in South Africa, in Torture and Its Consequences: Current Treatment Approaches. Edited by Basoglu M. New York, Cambridge University Press, 1992, pp 452–471

Emmelkamp PMG, Mersch PP: Cognition and exposure in vivo in agoraphobia: short term and delayed effects. Cognitive Therapy and Research 6:77–88, 1982

Emmelkamp PMG, Kuipers ACM, Eggeraat JB: Cognitive modification versus prolonged exposure in vivo: a comparison with agoraphobics as subjects. Behav Res Ther 16:33–41, 1978

Emmelkamp PMG, Brilman E, Kurper H, et al: The treatment of agoraphobia: a comparison of self-instruction, rational-emotive therapy and exposure in vivo. Behav Modif 10:37–53, 1985

Fairbank JA, Keane TM: Flooding for combat-related stress disorders: assessment of anxiety reduction across traumatic memories. Behavior Therapy 13:449–510, 1982

Fairbank JA, DeGood DE, Jenkins CW: Behavioral treatment of a persistent post-traumatic startle response. J Behav Ther Exp Psychiatry 12:321–324, 1981

Fairbank JA, Gross RT, Keane TM: Treatment of a posttraumatic stress disorder: evaluating outcome with a behavioral code. Behav Modif 7:557–568, 1983

Foa EB, Kozak MJ: Emotional processing of fear: exposure to corrective information. Psychol Bull 99:20–35, 1986

Foa EB, Steketee G, Rothbaum BO: Behavioral/cognitive conceptualizations of posttraumatic stress disorder. Behavior Therapy 20:155–176, 1989

Garcia-Peltoniemi RE, Jaranson J: A multidisciplinary approach to the treatment of torture victims. Abstract of paper presented at the 2nd International Conference of Centres, Institutions and Individuals Concerned With the Care of Victims of Organized Violence. San José, Costa Rica, November 27–December 2, 1989

Horowitz MJ: Phase oriented treatment of stress response syndromes. Am J Psychother 27:506–515, 1973

Horowitz MJ: Stress response syndromes, character style, and dynamic psychotherapy. Arch Gen Psychiatry 31:768–781, 1974

Horowitz MJ, Marmar C, Weiss DS, et al: Brief psychotherapy of bereavement reactions: the relationship of process to outcome. Arch Gen Psychiatry 41:438–448, 1984

Keane TM: Posttraumatic stress disorder: current status and future directions. Behavior Therapy 20:149–153, 1989

Keane TM, Kaloupek DG: Imaginal flooding in the treatment of posttraumatic stress disorder. J Consult Clin Psychol 50:138–140, 1982

Keane TM, Fairbank JA, Caddell JM, et al: A behavioral approach to the assessment and treatment of posttraumatic stress disorder in Vietnam veterans, in Trauma and Its Wake: The Study and Treatment of Post-Traumatic Stress Disorders. Edited by Figley CR. New York, Brunner/Mazel, 1985, pp 257–294

Keane TM, Fairbank JA, Caddell JM, et al: Implosive (flooding) therapy reduces symptoms of PTSD in Vietnam combat veterans. Behavior Therapy 20:245–260, 1989

Keane TM, Albano AM, Blake DD: Current trends in the treatment of posttraumatic stress symptoms, in Torture and Its Consequences: Current Treatment Approaches. Edited by Basoglu M. New York, Cambridge University Press, 1992, pp 363–401

Mavissakalian M, Michelson L, Dealy RS: Pharmacological treatment of agoraphobia: imipramine versus imipramine with programmed practice. Br J Psychiatry 143:348–355, 1983

Ortmann J, Genefke IK, Jakobsen L, et al: Rehabilitation of torture victims: an interdisciplinary treatment model. American Journal of Social Psychiatry 4:161–167, 1987

Rachman S: Emotional processing. Behav Res Ther 18:51–60, 1980

Richards DA, Rose JS: Exposure therapy for posttraumatic stress disorder: four case studies. Br J Psychiatry 158:836–840, 1991

Roth EF, Lunde I, Boysen G, et al: Torture and its treatment. Am J Public Health 77:1404–1406, 1987

Somnier FE, Genefke IK: Psychotherapy for victims of torture. Br J Psychiatry 149:323–329, 1986

Staub E: The psychology and culture of torture and torturers, in Torture and Psychology. Edited by Suedfeld P. New York, Hemisphere, 1990, pp 49–76

van Willigen LHM: Organization of care and rehabilitation services for victims of torture and other forms of organized violence: a review of current issues, in Torture and Its Consequences: Current Treatment Approaches. Edited by Basoglu M. New York, Cambridge University Press, 1992, pp 277–298

Vesti P, Kastrup M: Psychotherapy for torture survivors, in Torture and Its Consequences: Current Treatment Approaches. Edited by Basoglu M. New York, Cambridge University Press, 1992, pp 348–362

Williams SL, Rappoport A: Cognitive treatment in the natural environment for agoraphobics. Behavior Therapy 12:299–313, 1983

Yüksel S: Nature and treatment of posttraumatic stress disorder in torture survivors. Abstract of paper presented at the 2nd International Conference of Centres, Institutions and Individuals Concerned With the Care of Victims of Organized Violence. San José, Costa Rica, November 27–December 2, 1989

CHAPTER 9

Conceptual Models and Psychopharmacological Treatment of Torture Victims

Michael W. Smith, M.D.
Orlando J. Cartaya, M.D.
Ricardo Mendoza, M.D.
Ira M. Lesser, M.D.
Keh-Ming Lin, M.D., M.P.H.

For most of us, the horror of torture is inconceivable. Yet for those individuals whose incarceration has been motivated by political objectives, and for many prisoners of war (POWs), it is a cruel and savage reality. Institutionalized torture of political detainees alone has been reported in more than 90 countries across the world (Amnesty International 1984). Individuals fortunate enough to gain their freedom usually flee their homeland and seek political asylum elsewhere. Returning POWs and political

This work was supported in part by the National Institute of Mental Health Grant RO1 MH47355 and by the Research Center on the Psychobiology of Ethnicity.

refugees exposed to torture often require extensive medical and psychological care; the responsibility for providing this care falls to the medical and mental health professionals in the countries where they ultimately reside.

The magnitude of the abuse inflicted on many of these individuals can result in serious psychiatric sequelae, and pharmacological treatment is often an integral part of their comprehensive care. Accurate assessment of target symptoms is a critical first step in the selection of an appropriate psychotropic treatment regimen. However, psychiatric diagnosis and case formulation can prove to be a difficult and complicated process when it is victims of torture who are being evaluated.

In this chapter, we first briefly outline important assessment and diagnostic considerations in the evaluation of victims of torture. The section that follows is a summary of the existing data concerning the various etiological models that can explain the symptomatology manifested by these individuals. Last, we review the available literature regarding the psychopharmacological interventions used in the treatment of trauma survivors. Literature focusing on victims of torture is extremely limited. Scientific investigations into the area are hampered by factors inherent in the political nature of torture, by the victim's fear and psychological trauma, and by investigators' reluctance to deal with this highly charged topic. Because patients who are victims of torture share numerous similarities with patients diagnosed with posttraumatic stress disorder (PTSD), torture victims may well be diagnosed as having PTSD. Many of the data cited in our review of the subject, therefore, center on the research performed on patients with PTSD. To what extent the findings from the literature on PTSD can be extended to victims of torture remains unclear.

Torture Defined

The official definition of torture includes the following criteria: 1) the act constitutes a major trauma; 2) the event is one not expected to occur to anyone in a lifetime; 3) the act is intentional; 4) the pain and suffering are avoidable; and 5) the act is deliberate and is inflicted with the purpose of punishing or coercing the victim (Amnesty International 1987). The definition put forth by the United Nations Convention Against Torture and

Other Cruel, Inhuman, or Degrading Treatment or Punishment (1984) also stipulates that acts of torture must be carried out by or with the consent of a public official. Although methods of torture vary from country to country, the common denominator of humans' inhumanity toward each other remains. In a report on 319 survivors of torture from 15 different countries, Goldfeld et al. (1988) described various acts of brutality and violence, sexual assault, and deprivation. Follow-up studies have indicated that both men and women are victimized and that younger men as a group are tortured more frequently than others (Domovitch et al. 1984; Rasmussen and Lunde 1980). In addition to those individuals who have been directly affected by physical acts of torture, there are secondary victims who have simply been threatened with arrest or who have observed the torture of another, perhaps a family member (Cohn et al. 1980; Jones 1985; Ritterman 1987).

　　Certain unique aspects of torture are thought to be responsible for the complex psychological impact it has on its victims. Survivors of torture are not accidental victims of injury like victims of a natural disaster, for example. A torture victim receives the focused attention of an opponent whose task it is to cause maximum psychological change, usually by inflicting pain. Torture often is carried out behind the mask of a perverse intimate relationship (Ritterman 1987) and frequently includes deliberate attempts to disrupt normal healing processes, thus maximizing psychological scars (Turner and Gorst-Unsworth 1990). Furthermore, unlike other persons with PTSD, torture victims suffer a sense of personal shame and humiliation; a mistrust of friends, neighbors, and authorities; and confusion of values and self at the most intimate level (Allodi 1991). Allodi (1991) noted that the aftereffects in torture victims can be viewed as the direct result of the objectives of the torture: regression, humiliation, and confusion about the individual's values of life.

Obstacles to Diagnosis and Assessment

There are numerous factors that can make the assessment of and diagnosis in torture victims a difficult task. These factors range from issues involving the evaluative process to the content (sometimes highly affect laden and chaotic or disorganized) obtained during interviews to the multiplicity of symptoms to the restraints of our current diagnostic system.

Interviewing a victim of torture demands a special sensitivity on the part of the evaluator. Mental health personnel must be aware of countertransference feelings that can be evoked during the evaluation process and that may cause them to avoid details of the history and its emotional concomitants. Conversely, special care must be taken to avoid triggering reactions of fear, extreme anxiety, or painful associations to previous torture-related experiences (Allodi 1991). Interviewers should also be aware that in some countries medical and mental health professionals have collaborated in the perpetration of torture (Allodi and Cowgill 1982; Stover and Nightingale 1985; Vesti and Espersen 1990). In a study of 200 victims of torture from 18 separate countries, Rasmussen (1990) reported that 5% of victims confirmed the presence of a physician during the torture. In some of these cases, doctors advised tormentors concerning the continuation of torture. Such experiences would certainly complicate the assessment and the establishment of a therapeutic alliance and affect compliance with treatment plans.

Other factors also may be involved in determining therapeutic outcome. Lindy et al. (1981) explored the effectiveness of outreach efforts in individuals who had recently endured a severe psychological trauma. The results of their work and that of others (Poulshock and Cohen 1975; Terr 1983) point to an optimal window of 1–3 months during which emotionally overwhelmed patients can most effectively be engaged in evaluation and treatment. After this 3-month period, people appear less willing to be evaluated in spite of active symptomatology. A variety of factors were suggested that could account for this observation, including intrapsychic issues such as the struggle of the survivors to seal out painful memories by avoiding treatment. Burstein (1986) reviewed treatment compliance in 59 patients experiencing PTSD. He reported that only 27% of patients entering treatment during the first 9 weeks after trauma discontinued their follow-up visits, compared with 82% of patients who entered treatment after the 40th week posttrauma.

Cognitive deficits have been reported in survivors of severe trauma (Goldstein et al. 1987; Sutker et al. 1990a, 1990b; Thygesen et al. 1970) and may hinder the initial gathering of information as well as affect long-term outcome if patients cannot understand or remember treatment guidelines. Sutker et al. (1988) compared the long-term psychological and psychiatric sequelae in 22 POWs with those in a control group of combat veterans not exposed to the severe trauma of being a prisoner.

POW survivors were found to exhibit significant cognitive deficits when compared with combat veterans of similar ages and educational backgrounds. The results of Wechsler Memory Scale and Wechsler Adult Intelligence Scale—Revised (WAIS-R) testing revealed poor performance on tasks that required memory, attention, and concentration.

Victims of torture represent a heterogeneous population exhibiting a variety of clinical features, commonly including depressive, dissociative, and anxiety-related symptoms (Carlson and Rosser-Hogan 1991). In addition to each of these symptom complexes, alcohol and substance abuse must be considered in the history and presentation of these patients. With regard to treatment planning, the presence of alcohol and substance abuse must be dealt with directly, before or in conjunction with the modalities outlined below. A detailed discussion of these treatments, however, is beyond the scope of this chapter.

Explanatory Models Regarding Symptoms in Torture Victims

Torture victims have multiple and changing psychiatric symptoms, but for treatment purposes it is helpful to understand these symptoms from both psychological and physiological models. More targeted treatment interventions may then be possible. We will briefly review a few of the models that are more useful in this regard.

Psychodynamic Theory

Freud (1920) suggested that a traumatic neurosis occurs after a trauma leads to a break in the stimulus barrier. The individual's usual adaptive capabilities are disrupted, leading to the use of a more primitive form of defense, the repetition compulsion, which consists of mentally repeating the disturbing event over and over. By repeating the trauma in dreams and while awake, the individual replaces a passive, victimized posture with one that is active and mastered. The concept of the stimulus barrier can also be understood to have a biological or constitutional component, somewhat analogous to temperament. Kardiner and Spiegel (1947) described chronic posttraumatic stress as a "physioneurosis," thereby calling attention to the biological component of the disorder and the fundamental alteration that can occur in the autonomic nervous system.

Horowitz (1976) has contributed greatly to our understanding of the psychological and cognitive aspects of the response to trauma. He emphasized the impact of traumatic events on cognitive schema and the role of controls (defensive functioning) regulating the processing of information. After the insult, two responses—denial and intrusion—occur. This repetition of the event causes feelings of distress that are controlled by the coping mechanisms of numbing and avoidance. The two states of denial and intrusion alternate and gradually decrease in severity and frequency until a new equilibrium is established.

Inescapable Shock, Learned Helplessness, and the Noradrenergic System

A well-studied paradigm, whereby experimental animals are repeatedly exposed to inescapable shock or trauma and then do not try to escape the shock even when they are permitted to do so, has led to the concept of *learned helplessness* (Maier and Seligman 1976). These experimental animals exhibit 1) evidence of chronic subjective distress, 2) deficits in learning to escape novel adverse situations, and 3) decreased motivation for learning new contingencies (changes in paradigms). This model has been applied to an understanding of depression and is also potentially applicable to PTSD.

Inescapable stress results in the initial mobilization and subsequent depletion of norepinephrine and dopamine, suggesting catecholaminergic mediation of symptoms in stressed animals. Van der Kolk and Greenberg (1987) have suggested that the negative and avoidant symptoms seen in victims of severe trauma parallel those symptoms in experimental animals associated with relative norepinephrine depletion. Intrusive and hyperactive features (startle responses, hypervigilance, explosive outbursts) may be conversely related to chronic noradrenergic hypersensitivity, which may follow transient catecholamine depletion after acute trauma in animals.

The locus ceruleus is the primary source of noradrenergic innervation of the limbic system, the cerebral cortex, the cerebellum, and to a lesser degree the hypothalamus (Grant and Redmond 1981). Massive trauma may precipitate a tendency to respond with excessive autonomic activity by altering locus ceruleus activity. Certain medications useful in treating

PTSD (e.g., tricyclic antidepressants and clonidine [discussed later in this chapter]) have been reported to prevent symptoms of learned helplessness in experimental animals when infused directly into the locus ceruleus (Davidson 1992).

Endogenous Opioid Systems

Animals exposed to inescapable shock or other chronic stressors may develop analgesia with reexposure to the stressor. This phenomenon seems to be mediated by the opioid system, because it can be reversed by the narcotic antagonist naloxone. Thus, chronic stress may result in a physiological state somewhat resembling dependence on opioids. Similarities between opioid withdrawal symptoms (anxiety, irritability, insomnia, explosive outbursts, hyperalertness) and PTSD symptoms were described by Van der Kolk and Greenberg (1987). A study involving combat veterans with PTSD showed that reexposure to a traumatic stressor (a combat video) precipitated opioid-mediated, stress-induced analgesia that was reduced with naloxone therapy (Van der Kolk et al. 1989), further lending support to the hypothesis that dysregulation in the opioid system may occur in traumatized individuals.

Endogenous opioids may be responsible for other emotional correlates seen in survivors of trauma. Such individuals frequently demonstrate a triad of depersonalization, physical analgesia, and emotional blunting or numbing. These features reportedly have been abolished by acts of self-mutilation and by administration of naloxone (Richardson and Zaleski 1983; Sandman et al. 1987). The success in reducing self-mutilating stress-related behavior through the use of methadone, naloxone, and clonidine provides further support for the relevance of opioid systems regulation in victims of severe trauma (Van der Kolk and Greenberg 1987).

Kindling

The concept of kindling suggests that repeated presentations of subthreshold stimuli can sensitize neuronal pathways, ultimately leading to a reduced threshold for neuronal firing (Post and Kopanda 1976). Kindling has relevance to clinical phenomena such as seizures and cocaine and alcohol withdrawal. In the context of PTSD, this model suggests that cumulative stimulation in limbic structures secondary to repeated psychic stressors can lead to neurobiological changes, making victims more susceptible to emotional reactions to subthreshold (e.g., nonthreatening) stimuli: dreams, recollections, or neutral environment cues.

Kolb (1984) suggested that many of the symptoms seen in PTSD result from a loss of inhibitory cortical control over structures involved in alarm and arousal such as the locus ceruleus and the medial hypothalamic nuclei. Sympathetic hyperarousal states may continue the kindling process in limbic nuclei (Friedman 1988), and this may explain how a condition such as PTSD can persist for decades or worsen over time.

Psychopharmacology of Torture Victims

As previously stated, research focusing on psychopharmacological treatment of victims of torture is severely lacking. It is apparent that many of these individuals suffer from PTSD, and the pharmacological treatment of this disorder provides a framework for the following discussion. Treatment decisions will depend on the individual symptom complex, and treatment may include a broad array of psychotropic agents. In addition, many victims of torture are members of ethnic minorities, and a basic understanding of the differential response to psychotropic agents displayed by various ethnic groups might serve to enhance response to medications and to minimize side effects.

Antidepressants

Tricyclic antidepressants. The efficacy of tricyclic antidepressants (TCAs) in the treatment of PTSD has been the subject of numerous clinical investigations. Several open-label studies have reported modest improvement of PTSD symptomatology in patients treated with TCAs (Blake 1986; Burstein 1984; Falcon et al. 1985; Kauffmann et al. 1987; Marshall 1975; White 1983). Certain PTSD symptoms, such as intrusive recollections, distressing dreams, sleep disturbance, and increased startle response, appear to show the greatest improvement in response to the administration of TCAs. In a recent study of patients with PTSD, Chen (1991) reported that intrusive recollections appeared to be particularly responsive to treatment with clomipramine, a TCA used in the treatment of patients with obsessive-compulsive disorder.

Additional support for the efficacy of TCAs in the treatment of PTSD comes from studies using a placebo control design. Davidson et al. (1990) demonstrated that amitriptyline in dosages ranging from 50 to 300 mg/day was more effective than placebo for the treatment of PTSD in World War II veterans and in veterans of the Korean and Vietnam conflicts. In a double-blind study of 60 outpatient Vietnam veterans, imipramine also proved more effective than placebo in ameliorating PTSD symptomatology (Kosten et al. 1991). In contrast to the previous findings, Reist et al. (1989) found no statistical difference between desipramine and placebo with respect to relief of PTSD symptoms but did note some improvement in depressive symptomatology. Therapeutic blood levels were achieved in all three studies; however, patients were treated for 8 weeks in the studies by Kosten et al. (1991) and Davidson et al. (1990) and only 4 weeks in the study by Reist et al. (1989). This difference in duration of treatment may account for the conflicting findings.

Monoamine oxidase inhibitors. The results of uncontrolled studies (Davidson et al. 1987; Hogben and Cornfield 1981) attest to the beneficial effects of monoamine oxidase inhibitors (MAOIs) on PTSD symptomatology. The strongest ameliorative impact of MAOIs, like that of the TCAs, appears to be on nightmares, increased startle response, and flashbacks. Two controlled studies have yielded mixed results. In a study of four Israeli veterans and six civilians with PTSD, Shestatsky et al. (1988) found no significant differences between patients treated for 5 weeks with 30–90 mg of phenelzine and subjects treated with placebo. Conversely, Kosten et al. (1991) reported differential effects of 60–75 mg of phenelzine, 200–300 mg of imipramine, and placebo for the treatment of PTSD in 60 Vietnam veterans. Phenelzine therapy was superior to imipramine therapy, and both were superior to placebo in improving the intrusive symptoms, such as nightmares, flashbacks, and intrusive recollections. In addition, phenelzine improved symptoms of emotional numbing and distancing from loved ones and actively suppressed memories of Vietnam. The variance between the two studies may be due to study design, sample size, duration of treatment, and medication dosing.

Selective serotonin reuptake inhibitors. A few clinical case reports have described the use of fluoxetine in the treatment of PTSD (Davidson et al. 1991; March 1992; McDougle et al. 1991; Moore and Boehnlein 1991). In one study (Moore and Boehnlein 1991), fluoxetine was used in the treatment of two Laotian refugees who were victims of torture and had previously not responded favorably to traditional TCA therapy because of severe side effects. Fluoxetine was both well tolerated and effective in reducing their PTSD symptoms, especially avoidant symptomatology. Although further research is needed, these early reports suggest that fluoxetine, and possibly other selective serotonin reuptake inhibitors (SSRIs), may be very effective agent for treating PTSD. To the best of our knowledge, no controlled studies have been performed using this psychotropic agent or other more recently marketed SSRIs such as paroxetine and sertraline.

Anticonvulsants

As previously discussed, kindling has been postulated by several authors to cause the persistence of untreated PTSD symptoms and the subsequent effectiveness of antikindling agents such as anticonvulsants (Friedman 1988; Lipper et al. 1986; Post et al. 1986).

Carbamazepine. In two open-label studies involving carbamazepine, a widely used anticonvulsant medication, modest improvement in specific symptoms of PTSD was seen. Lipper et al. (1986) reported on a study of 10 Korean and Vietnam war veterans suffering from PTSD who were treated with carbamazepine for a 5-week period. The results indicated improvement in intrusive symptomatology, hostility, and impulsivity. Wolf et al. (1988) studied 10 Vietnam veterans with combat-induced PTSD and described significant improvement in impulsivity, violent behavior, and angry outbursts after treatment with carbamazepine.

Valproate. Despite reports of strong antikindling activity (Post and Weiss 1989), only one open-label study of valproate, an anticonvulsant most often used in the treatment of absence seizures, has been cited with reference to the treatment of PTSD (Fesler 1991). In this study, 16 Vietnam veterans diagnosed with combat-related PTSD were treated with valproate. Dosing was based on optimal clinical response, and serum blood levels were monitored. Mean duration of treatment was 10.6 months. Ten of the 16 patients reported significant improvement in hyperarousal and hyperactivity, as well as significant improvement in avoidance and withdrawal symptoms. Patients were allowed to remain on other psychotropic agents; therefore, caution should be used in interpreting the results.

Lithium Carbonate

Lithium is believed to exert its therapeutic effect through a number of possible mechanisms, including interference with kindling (Goodwin and Jamison 1990), decreasing noradrenergic autonomic arousal (Van der Kolk and Greenberg 1987), and decreasing rapid-eye-movement (REM) sleep (Chernik et al. 1974; Kupfer et al. 1974). Pharmacological and neuroendocrine studies of patients with PTSD have shown increased levels of noradrenergic hormones, indicating hyperarousal of the autonomic nervous system (Yehuda et al. 1990) and sleep dysfunction (van Kammen et al. 1990). The results of these studies indicate that lithium may be beneficial in the treatment of patients with PTSD; however, the literature attesting to its use in this disorder is scant.

In an open-label study, Van der Kolk (1983) studied 14 patients with PTSD whose main complaints were frequent nightmares, increased startle response, and impending loss of control. Treatment with lithium produced improvement in flashbacks, startle response, anger, and psychological stress in 8 of the 14 patients. In an open trial of low-dose lithium in 5 Vietnam veterans, Kitchner and Greenstein (1985) reported improvement in sleep disturbance, concentration, startle response, and anger.

Benzodiazepines

Benzodiazepines are widely prescribed for a variety of anxiety states and responses to traumatic situations. Ciccone et al. (1988) reported that at a Veterans Administration clinic, 71% of 105 outpatients diagnosed with chronic PTSD received long-term benzodiazepine therapy as part of their pharmacological treatment (36% were taking only benzodiazepines). Although the study appears to suggest that benzodiazepines are widely prescribed in the treatment of PTSD, their efficacy has been poorly studied.

In an open-label study of the use of clonazepam in the treatment of 5 patients with multiple personality disorder and PTSD, long-term improvement in nightmares, flashbacks, insomnia, severe anxiety, and general well-being was seen (Lowenstein et al. 1988). Alprazolam in dosages of 0.5–6 mg/day was studied in an open-label fashion in 20 veterans with PTSD (Feldman 1987). Sixteen of the 20 patients reported improvement in sleep, anxiety, irritability, and autonomic symptoms, although 4 patients reported an increased frequency of angry outbursts. In addition, a double-blind crossover study comparing the effect of alprazolam with that of placebo in 10 patients with PTSD was conducted by Braun et al. (1990). Although improvements in anxiety symptomatology were noted, symptoms specific to PTSD remained unaffected.

Another study of benzodiazepines in the treatment of PTSD points out the complications that may be associated with long-term use of these compounds. Risse et al. (1990) studied eight patients (the majority of whom had preexisting dependence problems with alcohol or benzodiazepines) with combat-induced PTSD. These patients had been treated with alprazolam (maximum dosage of 2–9 mg/day) for 1–5 years and then the medication had been withdrawn. All had severe reactions, including symptoms of anxiety, hyperalertness, sleep disturbance, nightmares, intrusive thoughts, and rage reactions, and six patients reported homicidal ideation. This study highlighted the potential problems of using benzodiazepines in this population with histories of drug use and reinforces the importance of gradual discontinuation of such medications.

Buspirone

Buspirone is a novel nonbenzodiazepine anxiolytic that is used clinically to treat chronic anxiety, particularly when such anxiety is mixed with depressive symptomatology. Animal studies have shown that buspirone blocks the potentiation of poststartle activity in conditioned-fear responses (Munonyedi et al. 1991). Two studies of the use of buspirone in the treatment of patients with PTSD were found in the literature. Wells et al. (1991) performed a clinical study of three patients with PTSD. The patients were administered buspirone in a maximum dosage range of 35–60 mg/day. Improvement in symptoms of depressed mood, anxiety, flashbacks, and insomnia was reported in all patients, with a delayed onset ranging from 29–55 days. The second study (LaPorta and Ware 1992) noted clinical improvement after 2 weeks in two patients with PTSD secondary to emotional and physical abuse who were treated with buspirone (30 mg/day).

Clonidine and Propranolol

Clonidine, a presynaptic α-adrenergic agonist, and propranolol, a β-receptor antagonist, have been used successfully in the treatment of patients suffering from PTSD. In a 6-month open-label study by Kolb et al. (1984), the effectiveness of clonidine versus that of propranolol on PTSD symptoms was studied in Vietnam combat veterans. Of the 9 patients treated with clonidine (0.2–0.4 mg/day), 8 reported less explosiveness, 7 reported fewer nightmares, 6 had improvement in sleep disturbance, and 4 described diminished startle responses and intrusive thoughts. Eleven of the 12 patients treated with propranolol (120–160 mg/day) reported less explosiveness and fewer nightmares, 10 reported a decrease in intrusive thoughts, 9 noted improvement in sleep disturbance, and 7 reported diminished startle responses. Another study focusing on 11 children with PTSD secondary to physical and/or sexual abuse used propranolol in an on-off-on study design (Famularo et al. 1988). Significant improvement in scores on the Childhood PTSD Inventory was noted in 8 of the 11 children.

Recent reports suggest a possible role for clonidine in the treatment of patients with PTSD as an adjunct to TCAs. Kinzie and Leung (1989) performed a retrospective review of the pharmacological treatment of 68 Cambodian refugees diagnosed with PTSD. Data analysis indicated that imipramine therapy by itself was effective for 27% of these patients, whereas clonidine therapy alone proved beneficial in only 10%. However, the combination of imipramine and clonidine provided symptom relief in 63% of patients.

Neuroleptics

Several anecdotal reports indicate that low-dose neuroleptics are beneficial in treating PTSD symptoms in war veterans (Atri and Gilliam 1988; Ettedgui and Bridges 1985; Friedman 1981). Taken as a whole, these reports demonstrate that patients who may receive maximal benefit have the following symptom characteristics: ego fragmentation, poor impulse control, flashbacks associated with auditory and visual hallucinations, and impaired reality testing. Neuroleptics are known to decrease agitation, strengthen ego functioning, improve reality testing, and decrease positive psychotic symptoms; they therefore would appear to be an ideal choice for use in PTSD patients with the symptom complex noted above. However, research into the effectiveness of neuroleptics in the treatment of PTSD is extremely limited.

In a single retrospective study of 25 patients with PTSD, of whom some were treated with one of several neuroleptics as well as one of several antidepressants, 2 of 8 patients who received neuroleptics showed a moderate to good response (Bleich et al. 1986). Although neither of these patients was psychotic, symptoms of explosiveness, nightmares, insomnia, and hypervigilance did improve. The study design precludes making statements concerning the potential efficacy of neuroleptics in the treatment of PTSD, and further research is needed.

Buprenorphine

Buprenorphine is a mixed agonist/antagonist opioid analgesic whose utility has been studied in numerous psychiatric conditions, including depression (Emrich et al. 1982), psychosis (Schmauss et al. 1987), borderline personality (Resnick and Falk 1987), and substance abuse (Reisinger 1985). In an open-label study by Mongan and Callaway (1990), six patients with PTSD and other comorbid diagnoses such as depression and schizophrenia were treated with 0.15–0.30 mg of buprenorphine. Five of the six patients reported feeling less tense, hostile, and depressed and noted improvement in their ability to talk about painful topics. The onset of response varied from 2 minutes to 3 hours, and the effect lasted at least 6 hours. The majority of patients acknowledged a previous history of illicit drug abuse but denied current use.

Additional Pharmacological Considerations

Biological as well as nonbiological factors influence pharmacological responsiveness. The biotransformation of most psychotropic agents is dependent on liver enzymatic activity, protein binding, and certain environmental influences such as diet, nutritional status, smoking, and concomitant medications. In addition, social and cultural factors may influence compliance with the treatment regimen and may prompt certain patients to seek alternative healing methods. Researchers in the fields of pharmacokinetics and pharmacodynamics have demonstrated the impact of ethnicity on pharmacological responsiveness (Lin et al. 1993). Because of genetic influences, certain ethnic minority groups possess different forms of the various hepatic enzymes involved in drug metabolism and of the proteins that bind psychotropic agents in the bloodstream. For example, patients possessing a fast or slow form of the various drug-metabolizing enzymes for a particular psychotropic agent will exhibit widely divergent levels of this agent, leading to variability in degree of pharmacological responsiveness. Given that most victims of torture are members of ethnic minority groups, a thorough understanding of these issues is advisable for mental health professionals involved in the health care of victims of torture; these issues are extensively reviewed elsewhere (Lin et al. 1993).

Conclusion

Torture is an abhorrent reality of human behavior. Political efforts and pressures are needed to end this practice. Meanwhile, mental health professionals must be cognizant of its aftereffects and its treatment. This chapter has been devoted to a biological view of the psychological sequelae of torture victims and has described how an approach using biological and pharmacological principles may help ameliorate some of the suffering these patients continue to endure after the torture has stopped. No single approach by itself is adequate; pharmacological treatment can be successful only in the context of a healing atmosphere. When administered in such a context, pharmacological treatment has the power to bring great relief to patients, and there should be no hesitation in trying a variety of these measures. Clinicians should not become discouraged if a first-choice medication does not work; they should try multiple interventions until patients experience relief.

As is clear from the material reviewed in this chapter, many psychotherapeutic agents have been tried for the management of symptoms and sufferings of patients with PTSD, with varying degrees of success. Given that most of these findings have not been vigorously tested, it is difficult to make recommendations at this point. However, despite this relative lack of information, practical guidelines still are needed for clinicians working with these patients on a regular basis. Therefore, we suggest the following:

Patients with intrusive thoughts, hyperarousal, and depressive moods should be given a full trial of at least one of the TCAs. This should then be followed by trials of MAOIs or SSRIs. Although the study by Kosten et al. (1991) suggests that MAOIs may be more effective than TCAs, the use of these medications in refugees and torture victims may be more complicated because of the difficulties that are more likely to be encountered in these populations. SSRIs are not recommended at this point as first-line medications because of the limited experience with these medications in PTSD and the lack of controlled trials regarding their effect on PTSD. Given their favorable side effect profiles, SSRIs may prove to be a more rational choice for first-line drugs in the near future, when more information regarding their efficacy becomes available.

Patients with impulsivity and hostility as their primary symptoms should be administered carbamazepine, lithium, or valproate. Patients with symptoms suggestive of psychotic process or ego-boundary disintegration should be given low-dose neuroleptics. Although benzodiazepines have been used for the control of severe anxiety symptoms, their addiction potential dictates that these medications be prescribed only with extreme caution.

These guidelines should be viewed as tentative.

References

Allodi FA: Assessment and treatment of torture victims: a critical review. J Nerv Ment Dis 179:4–11, 1991

Allodi FA, Cowgill G: Ethical and psychiatric aspects of torture: a Canadian study. Can J Psychiatry 27:98–102, 1982

Amnesty International. Torture in the Eighties (Amnesty International Report). London, Amnesty International Publications, 1984

Amnesty International. Amnesty International Report. London, Amnesty International Publications, 1987

Atri PB, Gilliam JH: Comments on posttraumatic stress disorder (letter). Am J Psychiatry 145:281–285, 1988

Blake DJ: Treatment of acute posttraumatic stress disorder with tricyclic antidepressants. South Med J 79:201–204, 1986

Bleich A, Siegel B, Garb R, et al: Posttraumatic stress disorder following combat exposure: clinical features and psychopharmacological treatment. Br J Psychiatry 149:365–369, 1986

Braun P, Greenberg D, Dasberg H, et al: Core symptoms of posttraumatic stress disorder unimproved by alprazolam treatment. J Clin Psychiatry 51:236–238, 1990

Burstein A: Treatment of posttraumatic stress disorder with imipramine. Psychosomatics 25:681–687, 1984

Burstein A: Treatment length in posttraumatic stress disorders. Psychosomatics 27:632–637, 1986

Carlson EB, Rosser-Hogan R: Trauma experiences, posttraumatic stress, dissociation, and depression in Cambodian refugees. Am J Psychiatry 148:1548–1551, 1991

Chen CJ: The obsessive quality and clomipramine treatment in PTSD (letter). Am J Psychiatry 148:1087–1088, 1991

Chernik DA, Cochrane C, Mendels J: Effects of lithium carbonate on sleep. J Psychiatry Res 10:133–146, 1974

Ciccone PE, Mazarek A, Weisbot M, et al: Pharmacotherapy for PTSD (letter). Am J Psychiatry 145:1484–1485, 1988

Cohn J, Holzer KIM, Koch L, et al: Children and torture. Dan Med Bull 24:238–239, 1980

Davidson J: Drug therapy of posttraumatic stress disorder. Br J Psychiatry 160:309–314, 1992

Davidson J, Walker JI, Kilts CD: A pilot study of phenelzine in posttraumatic stress disorder. Br J Psychiatry 190:252–255, 1987

Davidson J, Kudler H, Smith R, et al: Treatment of posttraumatic stress disorder with amitriptyline and placebo. Arch Gen Psychiatry 47:259–266, 1990

Davidson J, Roth S, Newman E: Treatment of posttraumatic stress disorder with fluoxetine. J Trauma Stress 4:419–423, 1991

Domovitch E, Berger P, Waver MJ, et al: Human torture victims: description and sequelae of 104 cases. Can Fam Physician 30:826–830, 1984

Emrich HM, Vogt P, Herz A, et al: Antidepressant effects of buprenorphine (letter). Lancet 2:709, 1982

Ettedgui E, Bridges M: Posttraumatic stress disorder. Psychiatr Clin North Am 8:89–101, 1985

Falcon S, Ryan C, Chamberlain K, et al: Tricyclics: possible treatment for posttraumatic stress disorder. J Clin Psychiatry 46:385–388, 1985

Famularo R, Kinscherff R, Fenton T: Propranolol treatment for childhood posttraumatic stress disorder, acute type: a pilot study. American Journal of Diseases of Children 142:1244–1247, 1988

Feldman TB: Alprazolam in the treatment of posttraumatic stress disorder (letter). J Clin Psychiatry 48:216–217, 1987

Fesler FA: Valproate in combat-related posttraumatic stress disorder. J Clin Psychiatry 52:361–364, 1991

Freud S: Introduction to Psychoanalysis of War Neurosis. London, Institute of Psychoanalysis Press, 1920

Friedman MJ: Post-Vietnam syndrome: recognition and management. Psychosomatics 22:931–943, 1981

Friedman MJ: Toward rational pharmacology for posttraumatic stress disorder: an interim report. Am J Psychiatry 145:281–285, 1988

Goldfeld AE, Mollica RF, Persavento BH, et al: The physical and psychological sequelae of torture: symptomatology and diagnosis. JAMA 259:2725–2729, 1988

Goldstein G, van Kammer W, Shelly C, et al: Survivors of imprisonment in the Pacific theatre during World War II. Am J Psychiatry 144:1210–1213, 1987

Goodwin FK, Jamison KR: Manic-Depressive Illness. New York, Oxford University Press, 1990

Grant SJ, Redmond DE: The neuroanatomy and pharmacology of the nucleus locus ceruleus. Prog Clin Biol Res 71:5–27, 1981

Hogben GL, Cornfield RB: Treatment of traumatic war neurosis with phenelzine. Arch Gen Psychiatry 38:440–445, 1981

Horowitz MJ: Stress Response Syndromes. New York, Jason Aronson, 1976

Jones DR: Secondary disaster victims: the emotional effects of recovering and identifying human remains. Am J Psychiatry 142:303–307, 1985

Kardiner A, Spiegel H: War, Stress, and Neurotic Illness. New York, P Hoeber, 1947

Kauffmann CD, Reist C, Djenderedjian A, et al: Biological markers of affective disorders and PTSD: a pilot study with desipramine. J Clin Psychiatry 48:366–367, 1987

Kinzie JD, Leung P: Clonidine in Cambodian patients with posttraumatic stress disorder. J Nerv Ment Dis 177:546–550, 1989

Kitchner I, Greenstein R: Low dose lithium carbonate in the treatment of posttraumatic stress disorder: brief communication. Mil Med 150:378–381, 1985

Kolb LC: The posttraumatic stress disorders of conduct. Mil Med 149:237–243, 1984

Kolb LS, Burris B, Griffith S: Propranolol and clonidine in treatment of the chronic posttraumatic stress disorder of war, in Posttraumatic Stress Disorder: Psychological and Biological Sequelae. Edited by Van der Kolk B. Washington, DC, American Psychiatric Press, 1984

Kosten TR, Frank JB, Dan E, et al: Pharmacotherapy for posttraumatic stress disorder using phenelzine or imipramine. J Nerv Ment Dis 179:366–370, 1991

Kupfer DJ, Reynolds CF III, Weiss BL, et al: Lithium carbonate and sleep in affective disorders: further consideration. Arch Gen Psychiatry 30:79–84, 1974

LaPorta LD, Ware MR: Buspirone in the treatment of posttraumatic stress disorder. J Clin Psychopharmacol 12:133–134, 1992

Lin KM, Poland RE, Nagasaki G (eds): Psychopharmacology and psychobiology of ethnicity. Washington, DC, American Psychiatric Press, 1993

Lindy JD, Grace MC, Green BL: Survivors: outreach to a reluctant population. Am J Orthopsychiatry 51:468–478, 1981

Lipper S, Davidson JR, Grady TA, et al: Preliminary study of carbamazepine in posttraumatic stress disorder. Psychosomatics 27:849–854, 1986

Lowenstein RJ, Hornstein N, Farmer B: Open trial of clonazepam in the treatment of posttraumatic stress symptoms in multiple personality disorder. Dissociation 1:3–12, 1988

Maier SF, Seligman ME: Learned helplessness: theory and evidence. J Exp Psychol 105:3–46, 1976

March JS: Fluoxetine and fluvoxamine in PTSD (letter). Am J Psychiatry 149:413, 1992

Marshall JR: The treatment of night terror associated with the posttraumatic syndrome. Am J Psychiatry 132:293–295, 1975

McDougle CJ, Southwick SM, Charney DS, et al: An open trial of fluoxetine in the treatment of posttraumatic stress disorder. J Clin Psychopharmacol 11:325–327, 1991

Mongan L, Callaway E: Buprenorphine responders (letter). Biol Psychiatry 28:1078–1080, 1990

Moore LJ, Boehnlein JK: Treating psychiatric disorders among Mien refugees from highland Laos. Soc Sci Med 32:1029–1036, 1991

Munonyedi US, Arishikeshavan HJ, Shanbhogue RS, et al: Potentiation of post-startle activity by conditioned fear: effects of anxiolytic and anxiogenic drugs. Biol Psychiatry 29:683–686, 1991

Post RM, Kopanda RT: Cocaine, kindling, and psychosis. Am J Psychiatry 133:627–634, 1976

Post RM, Weiss SRB: Sensitization, kindling, and anticonvulsants in mania. J Clin Psychiatry 50:23–30, 1989

Post RM, Rubinow DR, Ballenger JC: Conditioning and sensitization in the longitudinal course of affective illness. Br J Psychiatry 149:191–201, 1986

Poulshock SW, Cohen ES: The elderly in the aftermath of a disaster. Gerontologist 15:357–361, 1975

Rasmussen OV: Medical aspects of torture: torture types and their relation to symptoms and lesions in 200 victims, followed by a description of the medical profession in relation to torture. Dan Med Bull 37 (suppl 1):1–88, 1990

Rasmussen OV, Lunde I: Evaluation of investigation of 200 torture victims. Dan Med Bull 27:241–243, 1980

Reisinger M: Buprenorphine as a new treatment for heroin dependence. Drug Alcohol Depend 16:257–262, 1985

Reist C, Kauffmann CD, Haier RJ: A controlled trial of desipramine in 18 men with posttraumatic stress disorder. Am J Psychiatry 146:513–516, 1989

Resnick RB, Falk F: Buprenorphine: pilot trials in borderline patients and opiate dependence, in Problems of Drug Dependence. Edited by Harris LS. Washington, DC, U.S. Government Printing Office, 1987, p 289

Richardson JS, Zaleski WA: Naloxone and self-mutilation. Biol Psychiatry 18:99–101, 1983

Risse SC, Whitters A, Burke J, et al: Severe withdrawal symptoms after discontinuation of alprazolam in eight patients with combat-induced posttraumatic stress disorder. J Clin Psychiatry 51:206–209, 1990

Ritterman M: Torture: The countertherapy of the state. Networkers, pp 43–47, 1987

Sandman CA, Barron JL, Crinella FM, et al: Influence of naloxone on brain and behavior of a self-injurious woman. Biol Psychiatry 22:899–906, 1987

Schmauss C, Yassouridis A, Emrich HM: Antipsychotic effects of buprenorphine in schizophrenia. Am J Psychiatry 144:1340–1342, 1987

Shestatsky M, Greenberg D, Lerer B: A controlled trial of phenelzine in posttraumatic stress disorder. Psychiatry Res 24:149–155, 1988

Stover E, Nightingale EO (eds): The Breaking of Bodies and Minds: Torture, Psychiatric Abuse and the Health Professions. New York, WH Freeman, 1985

Sutker PB, Allain AN, Motsinger PA: Minnesota Multiphasic Personality Inventory (MMPI)-derived psychopathology subtypes among former prisoners of war (POWs): replication and extension. Journal of Psychopathology and Behavior Assessment 10:129–140, 1988

Sutker PB, Winstead DK, Galina ZH, et al: Assessment of long-term psychological sequelae among POW survivors of the Korean conflict. J Pers Assess 54:170–180, 1990a

Sutker PB, Galina ZH, West JA, et al: Trauma-induced weight loss and cognitive deficits among former prisoners of war. J Consult Clin Psychol 58:323–328, 1990b

Terr LC: Chowchilla revisited: the effects of psychic trauma four years after a school-bus kidnapping. Am J Psychiatry 140:1543–1550, 1983

Thygesen P, Hermann K, Willanger R: Concentration camp survivors in Denmark: persecution, disease, compensation. Dan Med Bull 17:65–108, 1970

Turner S, Gorst-Unsworth C: Psychological sequelae of torture: a descriptive model. Br J Psychiatry 157:475–480, 1990

United Nations: Convention Against Torture and Other Cruel, Inhuman, or Degrading Treatment or Punishment. New York, Office of Public Information, United Nations, 1984

van der Kolk BA: Psychopharmacological issues in posttraumatic stress disorder. Hospital and Community Psychiatry 34:683–691, 1983

Van der Kolk BA, Greenberg MS: The psychobiology of the trauma response: hyperarousal, constriction, and addiction to trauma re-exposure, in Psychological Trauma. Edited by Van der Kolk BA. Washington, DC, American Psychiatric Press, 1987, pp 63–87

Van der Kolk BA, Greenberg MS, Orr SP, et al: Endogenous opioid, stress induced analgesia and posttraumatic stress disorder. Psychopharmacol Bull 25:417–421, 1989

van Kammen WB, Christiansen C, van Kammen DP, et al: Sleep and the prisoner-of-war experience—40 years later, in Biological Assessment and Treatment of Posttraumatic Stress Disorder. Edited by Giller EL. Washington, DC, American Psychiatric Press, 1990, pp 160–172

Vesti P, Espersen O: Ethico-legal developments as a consequence of medicine in the service of repression: acceptance and resistance: trends in ethics and law concerning the issue of doctors' involvement in torture after the Second World War. Nordic Journal of International Law 59:275–286, 1990

Wells BG, Chu CC, Johnson R, et al: Buspirone in the treatment of posttraumatic stress disorder. Pharmacotherapy 11:340–343, 1991

White NS: Posttraumatic stress disorder. Hospital and Community Psychiatry 34:1061–1062, 1983

Wolf ME, Alavi A, Mosnaim AD: Posttraumatic stress disorder in Vietnam veterans: clinical and EEG findings; possible therapeutic effects of carbamazepine. Biol Psychiatry 23:642–644, 1988

Yehuda R, Southwick SM, Perry BD, et al: Interactions of the hypothalamic-pituitary-adrenal axis and the catecholaminergic system in posttraumatic stress disorder, in Biological Assessment and Treatment of Posttraumatic Stress Disorder. Edited by Giller EL. Washington, DC, American Psychiatric Press, 1990, pp 116–134

Section V

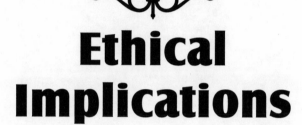

Ethical Implications

CHAPTER 10

Countertransference and Ethical Principles for Treatment of Torture Survivors

James K. Boehnlein, M.D., M.Sc.
J. David Kinzie, M.D.
Paul K. Leung, M.D.

Torture leaves devastating, pervasive, and lasting psychological effects on its victims. Moreover, psychiatrists and other physicians who treat torture survivors face a number of challenges, both clinical and emotional, during long-term treatment. During our treatment over the past decade of civilian victims of the Vietnam War and former American prisoners of war (POWs) who were subject to torture by their captors, we have seen highly emotional countertransference reactions in psychiatrists, other physicians, and health care providers of all disciplines.

Because medical and psychiatric treatment of torture survivors often involves politically sensitive issues, countertransference feelings frequently lead to ethical dilemmas. Should the clinician show anger and disgust at morally repulsive acts? Should the clinician reveal his or her own political beliefs? What if these convictions differ from those of the patient? Should the clinician encourage his or her patients to take political action? Should the clinician encourage religious activities for solace or atonement? How should the clinician deal with a patient's frustration and cynicism about a cruel world without causing that patient to give up hope or optimism? How may the clinician ethically handle his or her own feelings of sadness, frustration, or horror?

In this chapter, we describe some common countertransference reactions that we have observed in the course of treating torture survivors with posttraumatic stress disorder (PTSD), we offer some biomedical ethical principles applicable to psychotherapy and general medical care of these patients, and we suggest how these principles can be helpful for clinicians experiencing countertransference reactions during treatment.

Overview of Severe Posttraumatic Stress Disorder

Many torture survivors seen in clinical settings have chronic PTSD (Jaranson 1995). A knowledge of the features of PTSD is important to place countertransference reactions in a clinical context.

PTSD is a severe and often chronic disorder over which the patient has little control. The disorder affects many areas of the patient's life. The patient is not free to choose his or her symptoms, their development, nor the impairment that ensues. At the most clinically intense stages of PTSD, the individual suffers severe anguish, often has depression, and has a multitude of intrusive symptoms. These intrusive symptoms, which can have a variable course, often are greatly improved by treatment. A secondary series of behaviors includes avoidance, withdrawal, numbing, and estrangement from others. These symptoms respond less frequently to treatment over time and often become chronic. Treatment requires a coordinated treatment plan that includes biological, psychological, and social interventions. Results are frequently unpredictable, and patients can relapse even after periods of relatively good functioning.

Moreover, torture survivors frequently have chronic physical disorders due to the trauma, disorders that cause pain, functional impairment, and diminished self-concept. These results, in turn, contribute to countertransference responses from clinicians.

Countertransference Problems With Traumatized Patients

Since psychotherapy first was used in the treatment of traumatized patients, countertransference problems have been recognized and documented (Altshul and Sledge 1989; deWind 1971). We use the term *countertransference* to mean any and all emotional reactions a clinician has toward a patient, a definition that is consistent with that used by Altshul and Sledge. Countertransference is a multidimensional phenomenon that includes affective (guilt, shame, anxiety) and cognitive (fantasies, mental associations) reactions as part of an ongoing interpersonal process (Wilson and Lindy 1994).

Recently, a survey was conducted of the psychiatrists in our clinic, who have treated traumatized Indochinese refugees and/or former American POWs (Kinzie 1994). Among those questioned, there was surprising agreement about the major reactions that occurred within the therapeutic setting and also in the psychiatrists' personal lives. During treatment, most of the psychiatrists at one time or another experienced sadness and depression; anger, irritability, and a hyperarousal state; an excessive identification with patients; and intolerance of other patients with less stressful lives. Outside treatment sessions, there was an intolerance of all violence, particularly on television and in movies; a personal sense of vulnerability; occasionally a reminder of past painful memories; a sense of the failure of Western medicine and psychiatry; and sometimes even a sense that a culture that allows such violence to occur anywhere has failed. These were extremely broad and pervasive effects, ones that made a strong impact on the lives of the clinicians. Other researchers have noted feelings of helplessness and hopelessness among providers of treatment (Skrinjaric 1995).

In either the professional setting or in personal life, the physician who treats traumatized patients must normally struggle with his or her own intense responses. But beyond that, even a well-trained, well-controlled clinician faces moral and ethical dilemmas in dealing with the complex moral issues involved in treating survivors of torture. In this highly charged personalized setting, the ethical issues may become blurred as countertransference reactions take over. Recognition of these reactions is the first step in handling the ethical issues. In addition, it is helpful for the physician to have a structured ethical framework to help deal with the countertransference feelings that arise during the long-term treatment of torture survivors. In the following section, we discuss some of these ethical principles that can guide clinicians in their work with traumatized patients.

Ethical Principles for Managing Countertransference in the Clinical Setting

According to Beauchamp and Childress (1979), ethical theories can be divided into two major categories: 1) utilitarian (consequential) theories, in which the rightness or wrongness of the act is judged by its consequences; and 2) deontological theories, in which a feature of the act, not the act's consequences, make it right or wrong (*deontological* is derived from the Greek word meaning *duty*). This division has been further refined into holistic (deontological) theories, in which more than one basic principle is involved. Some basic principles applying to deontological biomedical ethics have come from the work of W. D. Ross (1930): the principles of fidelity, nonmaleficence, beneficence, autonomy, and justice. These principles are assumed, on sufficient reflection, to be irreducible acts that are held to be morally and ethically self-evident by any mentally mature individual. To these five basic principles, Thompson (1990) added the principle of self-interest.

We have used these six basic principles as our criteria for guiding ethical behavior in the treatment of severely traumatized survivors of torture, but clearly there are problems with this approach. The most obvious difficulty is that there are no clear guidelines when there is conflict between these basic principles. Also, in some respect, the principles are Western and not culture free; therefore, they are not universal. For example, for many Asian patients, autonomy is not a primary value and is not as highly valued as interdependence within a family and social system. Nevertheless, we have chosen these principles to guide ethical behavior because they are most consistent with our clinical impression of what is helpful and are also consistent with our ethical training as Western physicians.

Treatment of torture survivors involves a trusting, predictable relationship that often develops gradually (Gonsalves et al. 1993). Therefore, it follows that the most important ethical principle initially in the doctor-patient relationship is fidelity, which implies trust, honesty, confidentiality, predictability, and consistency. This relationship has strong therapeutic components (Haley 1974). In this relationship, the physician should not only be dependable and consistent, but also maintain his or her obligation to treat the patient over time. Yet patients sometimes are abandoned by clinicians for a number of reasons related to countertransference (Westermeyer and Wahmenholm 1989). The clinician, by being aware of his or her own affective responses, needs to recognize the ways that security and trust are communicated to patients. For example, because of the great emotional deprivation that torture survivors experience, the clinician cannot maintain complete emotional neutrality and then expect the patient to experience an atmosphere of trust, nurturance, and healing. Fidelity, as the paramount value at the beginning of the therapeutic relationship, encourages dependency over autonomy during the initial stages of treatment.

The second ethical principle, especially important early in the relationship, is nonmaleficence. Patients have already been harmed, deceived, brutalized, and traumatized in an unpredictable, arbitrary manner. It is therefore important that the clinician do no harm, which includes contributing in any way to the patient's sense of betrayal or vulnerability. As previously stated, it can be initially quite difficult for many torture survivors to trust their physician. Obviously, this will be particularly difficult if medical personnel were involved in the patient's torture. The patient may also fear even routine medical procedures, a reaction that may cause the clinician to become impatient or frustrated. The clinician needs to be calm and allow the doctor-patient relationship to develop gradually over time.

Therapeutic problems can take several forms, such as insensitivity to the suffering of patients. Through insensitivity, the clinician minimizes and trivializes patients' difficulties or pushes patients to get better faster than they are able. Telling patients simply to forget the past is also a harmful tactic, because it further trivializes their problems.

On the other hand, overidentifying with the hopelessness and helplessness of a patient and his or her personal remembrance of horrifying experiences may cause harm by preventing the clinician from recognizing a patient's strengths or from listening to essential personal accounts of a patient's life history. Danieli (1984) has described the "conspiracy of silence" by therapists who avoid talking with patients about their problems.

But another valid point of view is that therapists may feel that patients will be harmed by further self-disclosure; or therapists may recognize their patients' current need to avoid discussing painful experiences. The clinician walks a fine line between therapeutic distance and emotional neutrality on the one hand and emotional overinvolvement on the other.

Another possible source of therapeutic problems is use of a single therapeutic model, that is, requiring all tortured patients to talk about the trauma and reexperience the affect involved. The physician may unwittingly re-create the sadistic torture environment by requiring disclosure of painful experiences. This is particularly apt to occur in the early stages of evaluation and treatment before the establishment of trust and the development of effective verbal and nonverbal communication patterns that help to set personal boundaries within the therapeutic relationship. Because torture aims to destroy personal identity and integrity, the survivor often will have a heightened sensitivity to any infringement on interpersonal boundaries. Attention by the physician to these boundary issues from the very start of treatment can help the patient achieve one of the essential goals of treatment: the rebuilding of trust and security in interpersonal relationships. Additionally, some survivors will require lifelong treatment for the physical sequelae of torture, so it is vitally important that they be able to trust physicians.

We realize that the two principles of fidelity and nonmaleficence initially keep therapy cautious and conservative, limiting the physician's expressions and comments that deviate from a position of neutrality. This constraint puts strong demands on the clinician to maintain control of countertransference feelings until fidelity has been established, including finding ways to minimize any further harm to the patient.

A third principle, beneficence, is related to the physician's obligation to provide competent care and treatment. The goal of competent treatment is to reduce suffering and promote health, using treatment based on a sound scientific foundation. Lack of a scientific foundation leads to theoretical approaches that may not be beneficial to the patient and are not subject to scientific scrutiny.

A fourth ethical principle, autonomy, involves respecting and encouraging a patient's independence. With autonomy, the patient becomes a more active partner in the treatment program and begins to negotiate with the physician about personal goals and active participation in treatment. The patient is encouraged to explore alternative paths to health, to feel freer to take action regarding past wrongs against him or her, to obtain information, to read, and to discuss his or her feelings with others and with the physician. Further, the patient is encouraged to increase his or her involvement in relevant political, cultural, and social networks (Arenas and Steen 1994). He or she may choose to reestablish religious ties or may choose not to do so. At this point in therapy, the patient is less dependent on the physician and the physician is also freer in the relationship. For example, the clinician can share appropriate sadness and anger about what has happened and can perhaps even share political viewpoints, especially when they are sympathetic to the patient's cause.

The clinician should also be prepared to experience some feelings of sadness and loss when the patient grows away from the therapeutic relationship as he or she gradually gains autonomy. Because of the long-term nature of treatment after torture, strong therapeutic bonds frequently are forged, bonds that lessen as the patient rebuilds his or her self-identity and sense of personal control. It is important that the clinician be aware of his or her own feelings so that the patient is not kept in treatment longer than the patient needs or wishes to be.

A more difficult issue is deciding the extent to which the clinician can share personal views that are opposed to those of the patient (the patient may desire to engage in countermilitary action or even illegal activity to strike out against past wrongs, for example). The clinician must be particularly aware of countertransference feelings at this time so that he or she does not unconsciously encourage the patient to act in a particular way, thus compromising the very ethical principles that form the foundations for treatment.

At this point in treatment, the basic principle of justice should apply; for example, the physician may show justified indignation with regard to the wrongs the patient has endured or exhibit outrage toward the unjust systems that promoted such wrongs. The patient may be encouraged to protest the trauma of torture survivors by writing memoirs, telling personal stories to the press, becoming politically active, or even anonymously describing the traumatizing events in a public forum. Alternatively, of course, the patient may be supported in not acting in protest because his or her clinical condition—numbing, withdrawal, avoidance, or intrusive symptoms—may worsen.

Also at this stage of treatment, the clinician's cumulative reactions to treating traumatized patients should be considered. Here the principle of self-interest applies. The clinician may need to limit the number of traumatized patients treated, limit exposure to vicarious violence in movies and television, or seek support from colleagues. There also may be a need for the clinician to become more politically active and protest human rights violations that cause great physical and emotional harm. In this way, countertransference can be used as a medium for social change (Agger and Jensen 1994). The clinician may become involved in group advocacy or may support organizations that revile torture, such as Amnesty International or Physicians for Human Rights. The clinician may also volunteer for political activities and actively promote international peace and social justice. Just as important, however, are the personal means by which the clinician renews his or her interest, commitment, and, above all, endurance. These may include nurturing interpersonal relationships with family or friends, attending retreats, reactivating religious commitments, or engaging in recreational and social activities. The clinician does not leave therapeutic sessions unaffected, so there needs to be some self-interest in promoting his or her own security and safety and in nurturing of hope.

Finally, it is important for us as world citizens to bring the harmful effects of political torture to society's attention. If the clinician believes that he or she can speak on behalf of justice, equality, and peace and has the skill and means to do so, such action may be compelling, timely, and, above all, renewing of spirit and commitment.

Challenges for the Clinician

In the ongoing treatment of torture survivors, patients' stories are often emotionally distressing and frightening. They trigger anger and are even physiologically arousing. The therapeutic results are often frustratingly slow, and frequent setbacks occur. The clinician needs personal maturity and experience to keep the treatment on track. Even so, the countertransference feelings that develop must be constantly monitored so that the clinician can serve the therapeutic needs of the patient.

Regardless of the source of the countertransference feelings, it is helpful to keep in mind the ethical principles described earlier as means of managing those feelings. No matter who is the patient or what concerns are brought to therapy, the physician must remain constantly aware that the patient is a human being who is struggling with complex existential concerns regarding good and evil.

Because clinicians can be significantly affected by countertransference feelings, they need to develop strategies to cope with these feelings in both their personal and professional lives. In the latter stages of treatment, the therapist may even hasten therapeutic healing and growth by gently stating his or her own conflicting opinions to patients, for example, an opposition to violence or retaliation for prior trauma. Clinicians may feel free to use general clinical information in speaking out publicly on specific political issues. (Of course, they cannot use confidential patient records; trust and confidentiality are the most important aspects of the therapeutic alliance.)

Moreover, ethics do not exist in a vacuum but arise in a cultural, historic, and personal context. These principles serve as the basis for secure, albeit somewhat conservative, guidelines within an emotional and moral therapeutic minefield and help affirm the commitment of patient and clinician to each other.

The Medical Profession and Society: Preventing Use of Torture

Working with torture survivors over a long period and dealing with countertransference feelings often lead the physician to confront his or her own social role as healer and the medical profession's role internationally in either contributing to or preventing political torture. Torture unfortunately represents the medicalization of governmental power to abuse, maim, and intimidate. Physicians' skills and procedures are often used to carry out governmental mandates that directly contradict established medical practice.

In traditional world cultures, medical healers have been (and still are) viewed with trust and respect, the explicit expectation being that the physician cures illness and preserves life. In a disturbing number of developed societies, however, medical knowledge and procedures have been (and still are) used to destroy life. Prominent examples of the systematic use of torture by governments employing medical technology and personnel include the Jewish Holocaust, "special psychiatric hospitals" in the former Soviet Union, and atrocities by recent Chilean and

South African governments (Nightingale and Stover 1986). Physicians are no longer seen exclusively as healers and patient advocates, and this reduces the moral stature of the medical profession. This also greatly affects the torture survivor's ability to develop trust in physicians after the trauma.

Psychiatrists and other physicians who treat torture survivors must be acutely aware, then, of their own feelings when they encounter the devastating psychological and physical aftermath of medical procedures being used to dehumanize and maim. A broad perspective on the profession's standards and values can allow the physician to speak out effectively when medical knowledge and skills are being used inappropriately to carry out social policy.

One must continue to explore and critically question the foundations of one's personal and professional values throughout one's education and practice. If one does not, disturbing social trends such as the medicalization of torture can be accompanied by professional apathy or complicity.

Summary

The treatment of torture survivors is a long, draining process that often produces strong countertransference reactions. It is therapeutically and ethically difficult to handle these personal responses. We believe that at different stages in treatment, different ethical principles should guide the therapy. In the early stages, fidelity and nonmaleficence should be the guiding principles. As trust and confidence develop, clinicians may have more personal freedom to act; beneficence, that is, providing specific, confident care, then becomes the primary ethical principle. In later stages of treatment, the principles of autonomy and justice come into play. As treatment further progresses, the clinician's own needs, the principle of self-interest, may be used in the therapeutic relationship. Throughout therapeutic contacts with survivors of torture, the clinician needs to monitor his or her own needs and find appropriate ways outside treatment to cope with these often intense feelings. Continuing to feel therapeutically competent and ethically grounded, while maintaining the personal strength and balance to treat these patients, is a major challenge for the psychiatrist and the general physician.

References

Agger I, Jensen SB: Determinant factors for countertransference reactions under state terrorism, in Countertransference in the Treatment of PTSD. Edited by Wilson JP, Lindy JD. New York, Guilford Press, 1994, pp 263–287

Altshul VA, Sledge WH: Countertransference problems, in Review of Psychiatry, Vol 8. Edited by Tasman A, Hale RE, Frances AJ. Washington, DC, American Psychiatric Press, 1989

Arenas JG, Steen P: Exile psychology and psychotherapy with refugees in a transcultural perspective. Torture 4:50–53, 1994

Beauchamp TL, Childress JF: Principles of Biomedical Ethics. New York, Oxford University Press, 1979

Danieli Y: Psychotherapists' participation in the conspiracy of silence about the Holocaust. Psychoanalytic Psychology 1:23–42, 1984

deWind E: Psychotherapy after traumatization caused by persecution. International Psychiatric Clinics 8:93–114, 1971

Gonsalves CJ, Torres TA, Fischman Y, et al: The theory of torture and the treatment of its survivors: an intervention model. J Trauma Stress 6:351–365, 1993

Haley SA: When the patient reports atrocities. Arch Gen Psychiatry 30:191–196, 1974

Jaranson J: Governmental torture: status of the rehabilitation movement. Transcultural Psychiatric Research Review 32:253–286, 1995

Kinzie JD: Countertransference in treatment of Southeast Asian refugees, in Countertransference in the Treatment of PTSD. Edited by Wilson JP, Lindy J. New York, Guilford Press, 1994, pp 249–262

Nightingale EO, Stover E: A question of conscience—physicians in defense of human rights. JAMA 255:2794–2797, 1986

Ross WD: The Right and the Good. Oxford, Clarendon Press, 1930

Skrinjaric J: Ventilation, intervision, supervision, in Psychosocial Help to War Victims: Women Refugees and Their Families From Bosnia and Herzegovina and Croatia. Edited by Arcel LT, Folnegovic-Smalc V, Kozaric-Kovacic D, et al. Copenhagen, International Rehabilitation and research Center for Torture Victims, 1995

Thompson A: Guide to Ethical Practice in Psychotherapy. New York, Wiley, 1990

Westermeyer J, Wahmenholm K: Assessing the victimized psychiatric patient. Hospital and Community Psychiatry 40:245–249, 1989

Wilson JP, Lindy JD: Empathic strain and countertransference, in Countertransference in the Treatment of PTSD. Edited by Wilson JP, Lindy JD. New York, Guilford Press, 1994, pp 5–30

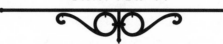

CHAPTER 11

Preventing the Involvement of Physicians in Torture

Peter Vesti, M.D.
Karin Helweg-Larsen, M.D., Ph.D.
Marianne Kastrup, M.D., Ph.D.

In trials after World War II, several doctors were found guilty of participation in torture. They were tried as criminals and were thought to represent a small minority of the medical profession. In the period after the war, there was continuous reporting of involvement of doctors in torture, but the issue was hardly accepted as a relevant ethical one before the 1970s. At that time, it was gradually realized that torture was still used worldwide and that doctors were not immune to pressures to participate. Today there are many reports of doctors involved in torture, outnumbering by far the reports of doctors involved in the pseudoscientific experimentation of the Nazi era.

One group found particularly susceptible is called *doctors at risk*. This term usually refers to doctors who are employed by authorities other than agencies and who have medical duties beyond clinical medical examinations and treatment. These doctors include prison medical officers, forensic doctors, police medical staff, and military doctors. Other groups of physicians may be included, such as psychiatrists and doctors working in developing countries. Doctors at risk are often professionally isolated and are thus more likely, at the request of authorities, to act against professional ethics. The doctors at risk may, however, simultaneously play an important role as witnesses of conscience—for example, by examining and describing lesions that are due to violence perpetrated in custody or by reporting inhuman treatment of prisoners.

Attitude of Medical Professionals Toward Torture

Different attitudes toward the problem of doctors' involvement in torture have been displayed. Some doctors find torture necessary to defend the country and have no objections to doctors being actively involved in the process. Others deny that torture exists and reject all the evidence, thus showing passive complicity. Some doctors have said that torture does exist but that it is a political problem, not a medical one. Many physicians have changed their attitudes during recent years and now regard torture as a medical and political problem. The problem of torture is increasingly described and discussed in medical journals, thus raising awareness in the medical community (Vesti and Espersen 1990; Vesti and Lavik 1991).

This chapter is an overview of the ethical foundation pertaining to doctor participation in torture. We review other primary and secondary prophylactic measures as well as tertiary measures that are taken to deal with transgressors individually and collectively, nationally and internationally.

Prophylactic Measures

Primary Prophylactic Measures

Primary prevention is based on the distribution of knowledge regarding torture to the medical profession through educational information.

Education concerning principles pertaining to human rights and medical ethics. The basic principle of human rights is that all persons have a set of fundamental rights that are inalienable. Concerns about these rights are relevant for all doctors in all doctor-patient relationships.

The aim of medical ethics is to guide the doctor in doing the right thing in a medical context. But what is right and what is wrong? Utilitarian theories such as universal act utilitarianism stress the consequences of any decision and state that it is adequate to choose solutions that benefit the greatest number of people, even to the detriment of a few. However, once such a sacrifice is accepted, perhaps even the torturing of a few individuals would be acceptable to save the many. This problem is often referred to as the *Manhattan syndrome*. The illustrative situation is as follows: a terrorist has placed a nuclear device in Manhattan, is caught by the police, but refuses to reveal the whereabouts of the bomb, which will go off in a few hours. Is it justifiable to torture the terrorist to obtain the necessary information and serve the public good?

Utilitarian principles state that we must be painstakingly aware of the consequences of our actions. Deontology, on the other hand, stresses that certain principles must never be violated. These categorical imperatives include not participating in torture, executions, or humiliating treatment of patients.

Categorical imperatives have been formulated for doctors through the centuries. They were first formulated in ancient Greece, in the Hippocratic oath, by which doctors today still swear to uphold the sanctity of the physician's responsibilities to patients. This oath states, "I will never do harm to anyone."

Any ethical consideration, however, must always be based on the concept of humans as rational beings with free will. The supreme moral principle is respect for the dignity and integrity of the individual, the right to make decisions, the right to choose norms and beliefs, and the right freely to express one's will. The autonomy of the individual is then violated if medical treatment or clinical trials are not based on fully informed consent. Medical paternalism might respect fundamental human rights principles, but such attitudes risk diminishing the autonomy of the individual patient and facilitating disrespect for ethical obligations.

The aim of the United Nations' Principles of Medical Ethics (Amnesty International 1984) is to strengthen the resistance against any participation in violations of human rights. They emphasize that any doctor has the right to refuse to perform duties that go against his or her conscience.

Yet further support for doctors facing the ethical dilemma of involvement in torture may be necessary.

Appropriate treatment.   The concept of treatment is generally visualized along an axis. At one extreme is torture and at the other is excellent treatment. In the middle is cruel, inhuman, and degrading treatment or punishment. Although a relatively clear concept of torture has gradually emerged, many gray areas have appeared, particularly concerning inhuman and degrading treatment and punishment. The most widely used definition of torture for medical doctors is found in the Declaration of Tokyo (1975), which states: "For the purpose of this declaration, torture is defined as the deliberate, systematic, or wanton infliction of physical or mental suffering by one or more persons, acting alone or on the orders of any authority, to force another person to yield information, to make a confession, or for any other reason" (p. 87). It has been realized, during the last decades, that definitions are often twisted by the authorities to avoid accusations of torture. Therefore, later conventions and declarations avoid definitions altogether; the European Convention for the Prevention of Torture and Inhuman or Degrading Treatment or Punishment (1989) is an example. However, the European Commission of Human Rights (1983) defined inhuman treatment, degrading treatment, and degrading punishment as follows:

> Inhuman treatment: Treatment is inhuman if it deliberately causes severe mental or physical suffering.
> Inhuman punishment: Punishment is inhuman if it is disproportionate and unreasonably prejudicial to the personal rights of the individual. There must be a reasonable relationship between the quantity of guilt and the opprobriousness of the crime on the one hand, and the punishment to be inflicted, together with its secondary consequences, on the other; punishment is inhuman if there is an intolerable disproportion between cause and effect.
> Degrading treatment: Treatment is degrading if it grossly humiliates the individual before others, or drives him to act against his will or conscience, or if it arouses in the victim feelings of fear, anguish, and inferiority capable of humiliating and debasing him and possibly breaking his physical and moral resistance.
> Degrading punishment: Punishment is degrading if the victim is hu-

miliated in his own eyes, even if not in the eyes of others; the humiliation or debasement involved must be other than the usual element of humiliation inherent in any judicial punishment; it does not cease to be degrading just because it is believed to be, or actually is, an effective deterrent or aid to crime control. (pp. 788–794)

Pregraduate medical education. Although the United Nations Convention Against Torture and Other Cruel, Inhuman, or Degrading Treatment or Punishment (United Nations 1989), Article 10, demands it, teaching medical students about the ethical issues relating to torture and doctor participation in torture has been endorsed by few medical schools and is not obligatory in the pregraduate training of physicians except in Scandinavian countries (Sørensen and Vesti 1990).

Other approaches have been outlined but never implemented (e.g., screening medical school applicants for moral defects and attacking the hierarchical structure of medical training. It has been claimed, for example, that the price for the current way of training doctors is a learned suppression of critical habits of mind, with the subsequent danger of subordinating one's own notions of right and wrong when they are contrary to the ideas of the prevailing society (Hofmann 1975; Jewett 1978).

Education of doctors at risk. Postgraduate courses in medical ethics and human rights have been initiated to strengthen the awareness about the rights of detainees. However, very few countries arrange postgraduate courses for the group of doctors at risk, although this is contrary to the directives of the United Nations Convention Against Torture (United Nations 1989). Such courses might be offered for all young medical doctors who function as military physicians, forensic scientists, medical health inspectors, and prison medical officers. The aims of such education would be to give the individual doctor the ability to identify ethical dilemmas in concrete situations, to identify special medical ethical problems, to recognize his or her personal ethical background, to aim at ethically acceptable solutions to medical ethical dilemmas, and to recognize a need for counseling in ethical matters if such a need arises; to instill in the doctor a knowledge of the relevant conventions of human rights and medical ethical principles; and to produce an awareness of the sanctions that might result if the principles of the conventions are violated.

Nowhere has the need for teaching medical ethics been expressed more clearly than in a statement by the defendant doctor in the case in South Africa concerning Steve Biko, who while imprisoned had been beaten to death: "I did not know that I could overrule the decisions of the responsible security officer" (Bernstein 1978).

Secondary Prophylactic Measures

Secondary prevention involves the development of ethical codes, laws, professional activities, fact-finding missions, and public education directed at stopping the involvement of doctors in torture.

Development of ethics and law. Ethical principles and codes give guidelines for answering medical ethical questions. They do not, however, present solutions to ethical dilemmas arising from discrepancies between deontological and utilitarian principles based on the society's laws and social norms. However, there are a number of declarations and conventions to guide the doctors in doubtful or difficult situations. Founded in 1947, the World Medical Association (WMA) is the international voice of medicine, serving as an advocate for physicians' views in addressing ethical and scientific problems. For example, the WMA Declaration of Geneva (1948) (World Medical Association 1970) states, "I will not use my medical knowledge contrary to the laws of humanity" (p. 330), and the International Code of Medical Ethics (World Medical Association 1948/1983) emphasizes that a physician shall be dedicated to providing competent medical care with compassion and respect for human dignity.

Adoption of national codes of ethics. National codes of ethics have a common background in the Hippocratic oath. Based on the principles in the oath and the International Code of Medical Ethics (1948/1983), codes for professional conduct have been developed by national medical associations. These codes typically have a core of principles that need to be continuously updated and adapted to the present situation of the country. These situations may require the inclusion of international ethical standards into the national codes of ethics.

Development of international codes of ethics. The most important advances in medical ethics have been the Declaration of Tokyo (1975) and the United Nations' Principles of Medical Ethics (Amnesty International 1984).

The United Nations' Principles of Medical Ethics was adopted by the General Assembly in 1982 to strengthen the standards for health personnel, particularly physicians, to protect prisoners and detainees against torture and other cruel, inhuman, or degrading treatment or punishment.

Proposed amendments to the Principles of Medical Ethics stress the right and the duty of the individual doctor to refuse to assist in any form of torture or other cruel, inhuman, or degrading treatment of persons deprived of their liberty, thus offering the individual doctor support in a situation of constraint. The Declaration of Helsinki (World Medical Association 1976), adopted by the WMA in 1964 and amended in 1989, guides every physician in all biomedical research involving human subjects.

International legal development. Brought about through intergovernmental cooperation, the major legal developments are the United Nations Convention (United Nations 1989) and the European Convention (1989). In these conventions, the duty to teach torture-related ethics to professionals, including doctors, is stressed. A difficulty has been the amnesties afforded to perpetrators of all crimes, including doctor participation in torture, committed before certain dates in some countries (e.g., Argentina, Chile, Uruguay, and Pakistan).

Organizational involvement. Organizations not previously devoted to the field of human rights have also given resources to the issue. These organizations include the American Association for the Advancement of Science (Stover 1985) and the British Medical Association (1986).

In relation to the issue of preventing doctors from becoming involved in torture, the former WMA was unable to act constructively; today, no worldwide organization of independent medical associations exists. Regional organizations in Scandinavian countries, Canada, the United Kingdom, the Netherlands, and Jamaica have taken up field initiatives.

International meetings. By the mid-1980s, the issue had so increased in importance that international meetings of the medical profession began being arranged around this topic. Three meetings stand out:

- Doctors, Ethics, and Torture (Copenhagen, Denmark, 1987)
- Physicians, Ethics and Torture (Montevideo, Uruguay, 1987)
- The Medical Profession and Torture (Tromsø, Norway 1991)

International and national networks of doctors at risk. The professional isolation of doctors at risk ensures that a blind eye is turned to violations of human rights. The problems concerning doctors' obligations to the individual versus the legally regulated demands for assistance in compulsory examination treatment are not always fully understood by physicians working solely in clinical settings. International professional support networks can facilitate regulation of the professional ethical problems of the doctors at risk and support these physicians in their roles as witnesses of conscience.

Assistance to foreign medical doctors working in countries employing corporal punishment. Medical doctors working in Africa and Asia may be called on to attest that a detainee is fit for corporal punishment. Some of the home governments of these doctors support them by providing notes confirming that doctors are obliged to apply the same ethical standards while working abroad as they would at home.

Minimum rules for the treatment of prisoners. In 1955, the United Nations adopted the Standard Minimum Rules for the Treatment of Prisoners (United Nations 1956). Articles 22 through 26 deal with the duties of the medical officer, which include surveying the conditions of prisoners and ensuring human rights. Likewise, the Standard Minimum Rules of the Council of Europe (1989), Article 32.1, states, "[A] medical officer shall examine prisoners undergoing disciplinary punishment, including detainment, to test that the punishment will not affect the prisoner's physical or mental health" (p. 24). The punishment can be applied only if the medical officer gives written testimony that the prisoner will be able to sustain the punishment.

Solitary confinement during custody, in which the prisoner is wholly or partly isolated from other prisoners, may under certain circumstances be in violation of the United Nations Convention Against Torture (1987). Individual tolerance of solitary confinement varies considerably. Experiences from many countries prove that the requirements of the United Nations Convention Against Torture are frequently not fulfilled and that prison conditions are often extremely poor. It is also known that, frequently, either there are no medical officers in these prisons or the medical officers are not granted, or do not exploit, the opportunity to object to inhuman prison conditions.

Impartial medical service in prisons. The obligations of prison doctors to testify to the effects of harsh regimes and to improve the medical and general sanitary conditions in prisons are best ensured when the medical officers are not employees of the prison. An unbiased, neutral, and impartial medical service promotes respect for human rights and facilitates critical medical testimony when needed. In several South American countries, even the forensic scientists are employed directly by the military authorities or by the police. These forensic scientists have in some cases, under pressure from the authorities, falsified death certificates and omitted descriptions of important lesions in autopsy reports.

Dissemination of information to the public. The issue of physician involvement in torture may be mentioned in the press of nontotalitarian countries; even in countries still under repression, discussion in the press has been possible. For example, a newspaper article from Montevideo, Uruguay, in July 1984 was headed "Yes, it was you I was referring to" and included a discussion of the exchange of words between a doctor accused and doctors accusing at the Seventh National Medical Convention (Denuncias en la VII Convencion Medica Nacional 1984). The authors of a work on torture in Chile wrote about the involved doctors and the struggle against them (Puebla et al. 1981).

Tertiary Prophylactic Measures

Tertiary prevention involves the development of corrective procedures that are to be followed when physicians have been involved in torture. The involvement of doctors in torture is made clear by the hundreds of denunciations registered, particularly in South American countries (British Medical Association 1992; Stover 1985). In a study of 200 torture victims, doctors were found to be directly involved in more than 20% of cases (Rasmussen 1990). In another study, involvement was discovered in more than half of the torture episodes described (Vesti 1990). However, gathering evidence is complicated because of the clandestine and illegal nature of torture, as well as the circumstances surrounding it (e.g., the victim may be blindfolded, torturers may pose as doctors, the victim may be cognitively impaired).

Once a doctor has been found guilty, the consequences vary according to the national measures of control of medical conduct. Medical doctors are responsible before the general laws of society, but in addition, a section of the law of the country specifically concerns the right to practice medicine. In Western countries, this control is vested in a statutory body that is either part of the central administration or an independent institution. This body controls retention of doctors' licenses by evaluating the integrity of physicians accused of criminal acts. The medical associations, in contrast, are independent unions, and membership is voluntary. Competing medical associations may also exist. The associations may impose sanctions, the most serious of which is expulsion from the medical association, and possibly remit records to the penal courts.

▶ *Actions Against Individual Perpetrators*

Court decisions. There have been few court cases on this topic since World War II. In one such rare case, Dr. Dimitrios Kofas from Greece was sentenced in 1975 to 7 years in prison. After 3 years he was released and was expelled from the army but not from the national medical association. He still practices medicine (Amnesty International 1977).

Administrative decisions. In one case, after the death of Steve Biko in 1977 in South Africa, the licensing authority, the South African Medical and Dental Council (SAMDC), took away the license of one of the doctors involved, Dr. Tucker, chief district surgeon. The other doctor involved, Dr. Lang, was only reprimanded and continued his career as a district surgeon. The Medical Association of South Africa acknowledged only the findings of the SAMDC (van Es and van Gurp 1987).

Decisions by ethical committees in countries with national medical associations. The following event took place in Chile in 1979: A detainee arrived at court in severe distress. A medical certificate presented on request attested that the detainee had been physically sound when he had left the interrogation center. The victim died in the hospital, and the doctor who had issued the certificate, Dr. Fuenzelida, was expelled from the medical association, as was Dr. Cesar, who had examined the victim during the torture (Goldman 1985; Larrain 1987; Stover 1987).

Decisions by ethical committees in countries with regional medical associations. Uruguay was the setting of the decision described here. In 1978, the death of a detainee was ascribed to natural causes in a postmortem by Saiz Pedrini, M.D. An autopsy revealed signs of torture, and Dr. Pedrini was expelled from the regional medical associations after investigation by an ethical committee for both of the associations. Dr. Pedrini continued as a military doctor at the time in the United Nations peacekeeping force in the Sinai and is still practicing as a medical doctor (Bloche 1987; Goldstein and Gellhorn 1982; Martirena 1987).

Decisions by ethical committees of local branches of medical associations. In a case in Brazil, a prisoner committed suicide, according to the death certificate signed by Harry Shibata, M.D. A postmortem demonstrated signs of torture, and Dr. Shibata admitted during the investigation that he had never seen the body in question. He was expelled from the medical association, but as a government employee he could continue his duties (Shibata 1980).

Popular tribunals. The following occurred in Argentina: A popular tribunal addressed the issue of doctor participation in torture because the medical authorities and medical association were unable to perform the task. Three doctors in particular—Dr. Jorge Antonio Berges, Dr. Hector J. Vidal, and Dr. Julio P. Esteves—were investigated and found guilty, but the only consequences were that the doctors' names were published in the national press (Comité Para la Defensa de la Salud, de la Etica Profesional y los Derechos Humanos del Pueblo Argentino 1986).

International tribunals. In recognition of the difficulties in dealing with offenders at the national level under a repressive system, a standing international ethical tribunal has been proposed but so far is not in operation (Vesti 1990).

▶ *Actions Against Perpetrators as a Group*

Repressive governments control the legal status of doctors and may dictate their ethical standards as well, including the standards of doctors working in psychiatric institutions. In such situations, medical associations from other countries must exert pressure through international organizations. As an example, the former Soviet Union was forced to withdraw from the World Psychiatric Association (WPA) in 1983. Subsequently, the Soviet Union accepted inspections on site so that it could regain membership in the WPA. Reentry was accomplished in 1989 (Bloch and Reddaway 1977; Koryagin 1988).

Discussion

Medical doctors still participate in torture. Under a repressive regime, the judiciary and licensing bodies are inadequate to deal with doctors who are involved in torture performed in the service of the government itself. Under such conditions, medical associations alone, by means of ethical codes, have been effective in applying some form of sanctions on perpetrators. Yet many doctors are not members of these associations; competing associations may exist or the medical associations may be incompetent. All of this clearly points to the need for a system capable of evaluating acts according to ethical norms, independent of the local law. When compulsory membership in a medical association is unacceptable, licensing bodies could be made independent of the government. In addition to the national ethics committees, an international tribunal and reporting system are needed, as are increased efforts toward prevention. All tertiary prophylactic measures rest on a foundation of medical ethics; this area is evolving, as evidenced by the major developments after World War II.

Further development is needed, and it is particularly necessary to stress that health personnel, particularly physicians, have the right not to obey orders to perform acts amounting to torture or other cruel, inhuman, or degrading treatment or punishment. By involvement in any such act, health care workers are committing a crime under international law and are liable to punishment if, under the prevailing circumstances, it was possible not to obey the order.

Expression of international support for and assistance to health personnel who resist involvement in acts of torture and other cruel, inhuman, or degrading treatment or punishment shall not be regarded as interference in the internal affairs of any state. Dissemination of public information about the existence of torture and other cruel, inhuman, or degrading treatment or punishment and promotion of educational measures for all medical and law enforcement personnel and public officials to counteract this phenomenon are obligations of all states.

The medical profession's awareness of ethical demands seems to be related to some extent to the organization of the public health system. A national welfare system, offering the public equal access to health care and respecting the autonomy of the individual, may serve as a means of basic prevention of medical abuse. It also offers the possibility of impartial medical surveillance regarding violations of human rights. Principles of respect for the integrity and autonomy of any individual, informed consent in medical treatment and trials, and equal access to health care are fundamental elements in the medical ethical codes. Concern with these rights is relevant for all doctors, including physicians examining and treating persons deprived of their liberty or undergoing punishment. The removal of doctors from the torture process will not stop torture, but it will make it more difficult for the torturers.

With regard to torture, neutrality by medical professionals is not possible, and the removal of the doctor strips yet another veil of legitimacy from the surrealistic world of torture.

References

Amnesty International: Torture in Greece: The First Torturers' Trial 1975. London, Amnesty International Publications, 1977

Amnesty International: United Nations' Principles of Medical Ethics (adopted by UN General Assembly 12/18/92), in Torture in the Eighties (Amnesty International Report). London, Amnesty International Publications, 1984, pp 258–261

World Medical Association: Declaration of Geneva, Physician's Oath (adopted by General Assembly, World Medical Association, Geneva, September 1948; amended, 22nd World Medical Assembly, Sydney, August 1968), in Principles of Biomedical Ethics. Edited by Beauchamp TL, Childress JF. Oxford, UK, Oxford University Press, 1983, pp 330–331

Bernstein H: No. 46—Steve Biko. London, International Defense and Aid Fund for Southern Africa, 1978

Bloch S, Reddaway P: Psychiatric Terror: How Soviet Psychiatry Is Used to Suppress Dissent. New York, Basic Books, 1977

Bloche MG: Uruguay's Military Physicians: Cogs in a System of State Terror. Washington, DC, AAAS, Committee on Scientific Freedom and Responsibility, 1987

British Medical Association: The Torture Report: Report of a Working Party of the British Medical Association Investigating the Involvement of Doctors in Torture. London, British Medical Association, 1986

Comité Para la Defensa de la Salud, de la Etica Profesional y los Derechos Humanos del Pueblo Argentino: Proceedings of the seminar entitled La Tortura en America Latina, Buenos Aires, Argentina, 1986

Declaration of Tokyo: guidelines for medical doctors concerning torture and other cruel, inhuman or degrading reatment of punishment in relation to detention and imprisonment. World Medical Journal 1975

Denuncias en la VII convencion medica nacional: si, me referia a Ud. Jaque [Montevideo, Uruguay], July 27, 1984, p 4, cols. 1–4

Doctors, ethics, and torture: proceedings of an international meeting, Copenhagen, August 1986, organized jointly by the Danish Medical Association and the International Rehabilitation and Research Centre for Torture Victims. Dan Med Bull 34:185–216, 1987

European Commission of Human Rights: Ireland v United Kingdom, 1976. Y B Eur Conv on Hum Rts, pp 512, 748, 788–794 (Eur Commission of Human Rts); see Peter J Duffy, Article 3 of the European Convention on Human Rights, 32 Int'l & Comp. L.Q. 316 (1983)

European Convention for the Prevention of Torture and Inhuman or Degrading Treatment or Punishment (and summary of the explanatory report). European Treaty Series, 126, entered into force Feb. 1, 1989

Goldman B: Chilean medical college battling doctor participation in torture. Can Med Assoc J 132:1414–1416, 1985

Goldstein R, Gellhorn A: Human Rights and the Medical Profession in Uruguay Since 1972. Washington, DC, American Association for the Advancement of Science, Committee on Scientific Freedom and Responsibility, 1982, xi

Hofmann FG: Commentary. Man and Medicine 1:191–197, 1975

Jewett FS: Commentary. Man and Medicine 3:52–53, 1978

Koryagin A: World psychiatry: readmitting the Soviet Union (editorial). Lancet 2:268, 1988

Larrain FR: Doctor torturers penalized by their professional body in a country where torture is practiced (editorial). Dan Med Bull 34:191, 1987

Martirena G: Uruguay: la tortura y los medicos. Montevideo, Uruguay, Ba Oriental, 1987

Puebla J, Fuentes R, Arcos V, et al: La tortura en Chile de hoy: experiencias medicas. Santiago, Chile, Ediciones Huichape, 1981

Rasmussen OV: Medical aspects of torture: torture types and their relation to symptoms and lesions in 200 victims, followed by a description of the medical profession in relation to torture. Dan Med Bull 37 (suppl 1):1–88, 1990

Shibata H: Record on torture victims "falsified." Amnesty International Newsletter 10:4–5, 1980

Sørensen B, Vesti P: Medical education for the prevention of torture. Med Educ 24:467–469, 1990

Standard Minimum Rules for the Treatment of Prisoners, Committee of Ministers Res. 73(5), Council of Europe. Collections of recommendations, resolutions and declarations of the Committee of Ministers concerning human rights, 1949–87. 1989, p 24

Stover E: The Open Secret: Torture and the Medical Profession in

United Nations: Convention Against Torture and Other Cruel, Inhuman, or Degrading Treatment or Punishment, in Methods of Combatting Torture. Geneva, United Nations Centre for Human Rights, 1989, p 17

United Nations: Standard Minimum Rules for the Treatment of Prisoners in Human Rights: A Compilation of International Instruments, Vol 1. Geneva, United Nations Centre for Human Rights, 1956

van Es A, van Gurp M: Health professionals and human rights in South Africa. Leiden, The Netherlands, Johannes Wier Foundation, 1987

Vesti P: Extreme man-made stress and anti-therapy: doctors as collaborators in torture. Dan Med Bull 37:466–468, 1990

Vesti P, Espersen O: Torture—the need for an international tribunal to investigate individual doctors who may have been involved. International Journal of Refugee Law 2:612–619, 1990

Vesti P, Lavik NJ: Torture and the medical profession: a review. J Med Ethics 17 (suppl):4–8, 1991

World Medical Association: Declaration of Helsinki: recommendations guiding medical doctors in biomedical research involving human subjects. Med J Aust 1(7):206–207, 1976

World Medical Association: Declaration of Geneva (1948), in Declaration of Geneva; Declaration of Helsinki; Declaration of Sydney; Declaration of Oslo. New York, World Medical Association, 1970

Section VI

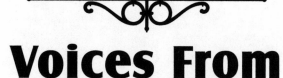

Voices From the Field

Politics and Caregiving

CHAPTER 12

Forced Disappearance
A Particular Form of Torture

Diana Kordon, M.D.
Lucila Edelman, M.D.
Darío Lagos, M.D.
Daniel Kersner, M.D.

Between the years 1976 and 1983, a military dictatorship established state terrorism in Argentina. During this period, the worst forms of political repression in the history of the country emerged. These were characterized by 1) illegal detention in clandestine jails and the disappearance of 30,000 people or more, the majority of whom were murdered after being tortured, 2) illegal detention in recognized jails of an additional 10,000 persons, also subjected to torture and inhuman conditions for prolonged periods, and 3) kidnapping of children and the changing of their identities. This repression led to the flight of hundreds of thousands of people who sought asylum outside the country.

After the military coup, executive power was misused and parliament was dissolved. A great number of judges were removed from their posts, and those who remained accepted the Statute of the National Reorganization Process, the postulates of which superseded those of the National

Constitution. Judicial power became subordinate to the decisions of the executive branch of government. In this period, the military granted itself immunity from criminal prosecution. No trials were held. In 1983, shortly before the first call for elections, the dictatorship granted a law of "autoamnesty."

When a massive popular movement reclaimed justice after the reign of terror, it brought about the first constitutional period. Three successive military juntas and some of the officers involved in the repression were placed on trial. Shortly after the sentencing of members of the military elite, two decrees (Punto Final [Final Point] and Obediencia Debida [Owed Obedience]) were enacted, relieving all of the accused of any responsibility (i.e., granting them impunity). During a second constitutional government, the executive office granted pardons and allowed the release of the members of the military juntas who had been tried and convicted. Though constitutional, the pardons endowed the president with a unique power, exclusive and independent of any social consensus. The pardon of those responsible for the genocide in Argentina was preceded by opposition marches of immense proportions. With the decrees, a system of exceptions and privileges was installed that challenged all judicial and ethical values.

The scope of the phenomenon of *disappearance* made it a paradigm of a junta's repressive politics. In light of its characteristics, we can consider disappearance as a particular form of torture, torture suffered by the disappeared and extending to their families and friends. The disappeared inhabited a no-man's-land, living beyond life and death, without legal protection, and at the mercy of captors. Family members had a high degree of psychological suffering and a profound alteration in their daily lives.[1]

To ensure social control, the dictatorship generated intensive propaganda campaigns. These must be analyzed in detail to understand the complex psychological phenomena produced in the relatives of the miss-

---

[1] In a quantitative and qualitative study of 50 cases of relatives of disappeared persons (L. Ricon, J. Braun, D. Kordon, L. Edelman, and D. Lagos, unpublished data, 1987–1989), higher rates of morbidity and mortality were found in fathers of the disappeared than in control subjects. In contrast, there was no significant difference in morbidity or mortality between the mothers of the disappeared and control subjects.

ing, as well as in society at large. Acts against the juntas were silenced. Although there were indications of and information about the existence of the missing, public acknowledgment of these facts was forbidden. The kidnapping of a son, friend, or neighbor, and then a permanent, formal denial of the event seemed particularly sinister. These situations were magnified by a total absence of information over many years regarding the outcomes of the disappeared. In spite of having previously been exposed to different forms of political repression, Argentinian society had never experienced such a magnitude of events. Many family members were unaware that a detention, even with its violence, could and often did lead to a disappearance or murder or both.

After a prolonged period of unsuccessful attempts to determine the whereabouts of their children, family members began to suspect that something sinister and previously unknown was occurring. These individuals were often prevented from revealing what had occurred lest they endanger their own missing. Many did not directly anticipate the possibility that their relatives would not return but understood that, in a larger sense, a system of political repression had been established in which the victims were "swallowed by the earth." An earlier repression of the indigenous population, accomplished a century before by the Argentinian oligarchy, used similar methods.

During the first years of the dictatorship, there was not even a term to denote the status of the people who had been kidnapped. Although it did not convey the violence or terrifying nature of the kidnapping, the expression *disappeared* was in time coined to state the destiny of the people so victimized. On occasion, some people who had disappeared were released. These people were threatened with death by their kidnappers to prevent them from speaking of the experiences they had had or of what they had seen or heard.

Reconstructing from the limited testimony available, the Argentinian public slowly came to know the immense physical and psychological suffering to which the disappeared were subjected. The existence of clandestine jails, as well as the terrible and sophisticated torture methods applied systematically to all the prisoners, became known. There were the so-called transfers, which in most cases meant murder and the disappearance of the victim's body. Large numbers of people received hypnotics and were drowned in the Rio de la Plata or in the ocean. This completed the picture of the atrocities implemented by the fascist dictatorship. The people of Argentina gradually understood. Information was transmitted by word of mouth, and organizations concerned with human rights began the difficult task of collecting data and denouncing these practices. From the start of the period of repression, families of disappeared members united as they encountered each other. They took steps to locate their relatives. Mothers occupied town squares attempting to demolish, with their public testimony, the walls of silence imposed by the dictatorship. Consequently, the movement Mothers of Plaza de Mayo was born.

Clinical Concepts

Trauma

The relatives and friends of the disappeared underwent a unique traumatic situation. We use the following definition of trauma: "An experience which generates, in a short period of time, a degree of stimulation to psychic life so extreme that it results in the failure of its extinction by normal or habitual means. This inevitably results in lasting alterations of energy function" (Laplanche and Pontalis 1972). This situation may be brought about by a single violent event, or it may be the result of the cumulative effects of multiple events, altering the psyche and the principles that guide psychic life. Forced disappearance constituted a traumatic event to the person involved and to his or her family and friends. Family members were usually involuntary witnesses of the kidnapping, which frequently occurred in the victim's house and involved considerable violence, theft, and destruction to the home, as well as beatings and torture of the victim and/or family members.

Despite the magnitude of emotional impact involved, we have observed in clinical practice a wide range of responses to these traumatic events, including nonpathological responses. We have witnessed active, adaptive behavior, even in people for whom these behaviors, because of various psychological and social characteristics, would seem unthinkable. Experiencing a traumatic event does not necessarily result in psychopathology; rather, a high degree of individual variability was noted. In the cases in which psychopathology did result, we observed a predominance of depressive symptomatology in the relatives of the disappeared. We also found a predominance of symptoms related to the repetitive reliving of the traumatic event in many persons who disappeared and/or were detained and then freed.

Laplanche and Pontalis (1972) defined traumatic neuroses as those in which symptoms follow an emotional trauma, one that is linked to a situation that threatens life or the subject's integrity. The trauma produces a significant number of the symptoms, which include nightmares, mental repetition of the traumatic event, and acute anxiety with significant somatic and neurovegetative compromise (palpitations, sweating, choking, and colic).

We have observed a diversity of symptoms in those we help. The following symptoms are the most frequent and severe:

- Mental repetition of the traumatic event—either as an agonizing dream (nightmare) with abrupt awakening and significant neurovegetative changes or as a reliving of the experience, triggered by an external stimulus linked to the traumatic event (e.g., sirens, the presence of military or police personnel, bells, or violent noises during the night)
- Avoidant behaviors related to the traumatic event: abandonment of activities and interests directly or indirectly linked with a traumatic event (e.g., activities related to or interest in politics or culture); often, the avoidance is reinforced by the realistic threat posed by the activities and results in abandonment of familiar gatherings and inhibition of social life
- Suspension or abandonment of vital projects; this phenomenon occurs very frequently and is directly related to the indefinite quality attached to the disappeared status; family members cannot go ahead with vital projects—for example, school, marriage, children—as long as the situation of their loved one remains undetermined
- Alterations in mood (anger, irritability, and rage attacks)
- Sleep disorders (insomnia and hypersomnia)
- Feelings of impotence
- Feelings of hostility
- Psychotic episodes
- Severe somatic disorders (cardiovascular disorders and cancer)

It is important to highlight the meaning of many of these symptoms, including their overdetermination and the role that social aspects played in their presentation. Here are a few clinical examples:

- The presence of a police patrol in front of the house of the parents of one of the disappeared triggered a flashback of the traumatic event in the victim's mother. It also constituted a real threat to the integrity of the family in the members' attempt to locate their child while risking their own lives.
- Those who complained about the disappeared, denounced the process, or even spoke about the subject were also at risk of disappearing. This generated alterations in mood and sleep.
- Social isolation and/or the abandonment of daily tasks or interest occurred as a direct result of the trauma but often as a result of the new tasks facing the families of the disappeared in the search for their loved ones. Some parents remained in their homes, awaiting the return of their disappeared children, a situation that became congruent with the social mandate of passivity and surrender.
- Feelings of impotence and hostility were observed frequently in parents, together with severe depression and serious somatic alterations. This seems to have occurred as part of an overall plan of social control through a systematic psychological campaign of blaming the victims and their families (Kordon and Edelman 1986).

For relatives of the disappeared, the trauma was of prolonged duration. Over a period of years, uncertainty regarding the status of the disappeared prevailed; then it slowly became apparent that the loved one had been murdered. This profound change from uncertainty to realization of the victim's murder represented a complex process not only for the relatives but for society at large. During the military dictatorship, some of the disappeared were alive in concentration camps, and people were obligated, officially, to deny the disappearance and/or death, despite much evidence to the contrary. Years later, after the end of the dictatorship and during the first years of constitutional government, hope of finding the disappeared vanished progressively as evidence of the assassinations emerged. During the dictatorship, however, assuming the death of the disappeared also implied accepting the dictatorship's rule. One must recall the military dictatorship's numerous psychological campaigns, which reinforced the pathological effects of the trauma (Kordon and Edelman 1986).

The theme of immunity from prosecution is important enough to deserve separate discussion. Those individuals ideologically and directly responsible for the disappearances during state terrorism are immune from prosecution even now. In our clinical practice, we have observed how each new political or legal measure that protects this immunity exacerbates, in many of our patients, the symptoms previously described. This process underlines the concept of social issues expressed through the individual. In the preface to "Psychoanalysis and War Neuroses," Freud (1919/1959) spoke of a self that defends itself against real danger, the danger of death that was present etiologically in these neuroses. In 1926, Freud (1926/1959) described the anxiety generated when individuals are confronted with an external real danger. A system of forced disappearance as a repressive measure peculiar to state terrorism clearly becomes one of those situations. However, besides the traumatic event per se and the psychological characteristics of the individual, the effective situation (Laplanche and Pontalis 1972) or the social circumstances and the demands of the moment play a significant role.

Bereavement

We conceptualize bereavement as the process that follows significant loss, involving either "a loved one or an equivalent ideal or abstraction" (Freud 1917/1959, p. 243), a process with the goal of working through the psychological suffering produced. The psychic process realizes the painful task of working through, which allows the person to establish the lost object in memory and regain an interest in the external world. The process of grief takes place beginning with the recognition of the reality principle, which, although initially rejected, eventually imposes itself.

In the case of a death, after a brief denial of the event, the psychic apparatus uses the reality-testing function, which allows it to discriminate between present and absent. It can then proceed to give the absence a sense of finality, attempting to adjust slowly to the necessary separation from the lost object. This process is termed *disinvesting an object* that previously was cathected.

In the case of transient losses, there is a similar process of disinvestment or decathexis, because the person who returns will not be the same, nor will the family or spouse. However, the certainty of the lost one's return is an indicator of reality; confronted with this, the individual can choose different options, as difficult as these might be. In cases of disappearance, however, a sense of uncertainty regarding the destiny of the disappeared is pervasive. The lack of reference points creates a state of severe ambiguity that is reinforced by the impunity of those responsible for the disappearances. This level of ambiguity prevents the reality principle from determining a precise direction for its work.

The normal process of bereavement initially includes rage, feelings of impotence, and resistance to accepting the loss. In the case of the disappeared, the family member does not know what should be accepted; this adversely affects the psyche, which confuses the therapist's elaboration of the patient's (the relative's) process. As a consequence, many therapists, also under the influence of the psychological campaigns of the dictatorship, have insisted that families accept the death of the disappeared as a condition of the grief work (Kordon and Edelman 1986). The dictatorship's efforts were to strengthen the perception that the victims and their relatives were to be blamed for the disappearances, and this reinforced the normal feelings of guilt that are present in all bereavement. On the other hand, the imposed silence regarding the disappeared, a silence that was maintained over many years, generated a situation leading to a social consensus in which the reality of what was happening was denied and rejected. During the processing of a death, the presence of the body is an important element that assists in overcoming the denial mechanisms. The role of funeral rituals is so important that we know of no culture in which they are not performed. In our clinical cases, there have been no death certificates, and no funeral rituals could be performed.

At present, the fact that all perpetrators of this genocide are free continues to aid the denial of the crimes. At the same time, the socially accepted freedom of the assassins essentially erases from history the existence of the victims. The freed assassins function, in a sociological sense, as a denial of the crimes against humanity. Every disappeared individual was thus made guilty. Every oppressor, as a result of the impunity, became innocent.

Faced with such a traumatic situation and its paralyzing ambiguity, the relatives of the disappeared, especially the mothers, generated a strong, organized social response. The emergence of this response had a significant impact on the grief process. Faced with the models and pronouncements generated by those in power, the mothers offered an alternative: a social and practical form of resistance and reality testing that brought back to public light the phenomenon being denied. The transforming power of reality had a direct effect on the protagonists of the social movement, but it also had an impact on the families and society at large.

In this process, the models that had been generated by the dictatorship and social consensus became increasingly recognized as such, and a gap was created in which other constructs could be formulated. Different social representations that acknowledged the version of reality that so far had been hidden and silenced could be generated. This social movement had a direct impact on the individuals processing the loss. Besides its personal, private, and intimate aspect, the grief acquired a public and social quality. With the generation of this antidictatorial social consensus, the necessary social representations were created to define the reality principle that would guide the process of bereavement. It was social consensus that produced public acceptance of the status *disappeared*. The disappeared now existed; the posters, the pictures in the streets, and the silhouettes created socially constructed reference points that supported the subjective representations. Individual psychic processes were able to use this social representation to accept the specific status produced by the disappearance. The working through of the bereavement process then followed this sequence: 1) searching for one's own child, 2) searching for all the children, and 3) demanding justice so that such a thing would never occur again.

Two Case Examples

The patients described in this section were treated at our facility.

Jorge

Marta, 54, and José, 56, had three children: Jorge, the oldest, who disappeared in June 1976 when he was 19; Guillermo, who was 23; and Estela, who was 18.

Until the moment of Jorge's disappearance, the family described itself as a "family like the rest." In our clinical view, Marta and José had maintained a significant sense of intimacy, an active sexual life, and good boundaries with their children. José was a well-positioned employee in a business. His job was highly valued by his family. He was described by his wife and children as being, until Jorge's disappearance, warm and strong, slightly irascible, and very responsible at his job. Marta was a housewife and had a part-time job. The three children were students. The family maintained daily contact with their neighbors. They had warm ties to José's family because Marta was an only child and her parents had died many years earlier.

At the time of Jorge's disappearance, the first emotional impact on the family was to make the family greatly concerned about what might have happened, and the family's belief was that he had been detained. The family members were not aware of the phenomenon of disappearance, and for some time the situation was one of anxious waiting. Every doorbell, any noise, heightened everyone's attention and raised the possibility that Jorge had returned or that at least someone had brought news about him. As they began to inquire and to contact official agencies, they became aware of the existence of many other cases like Jorge's. The idea that he might not return, however, did not occur to them. For some time, family life centered around anxious waiting; they had to be home in case there was news, and there had to be food in the refrigerator in case he arrived and was hungry. In the meantime, anxiety grew, particularly for Marta and José, who began to learn from other families about kidnapped people who had been subjected to torture and inhuman conditions.

The confirmation of Jorge's disappeared status created a situation of ambiguity. José suffered from severe depression during this period, believing he had not protected his son adequately and thus prevented his disappearance. Jorge's political activity as a student was well known to the family. José and Marta had suggested, out of fear, that he abandon his activism. José still blamed himself, using various and often contradictory arguments, for not having saved his child. His depression forced him, despite his wishes, to an early retirement because of incapacity. In addition, he was told that the fact that he had a disappeared child created a difficult situation for his company in the country's political climate.

José's depressive episode was well resolved after a few months, but by then he was a "retired member" of the household, which reinforced his feelings of impotence. During that period, Marta became involved in multiple activities aimed at locating her disappeared son and had to increase her working hours because of growing economic needs. Family members were no longer welcome in the neighborhood, some of their neighbors became mistrustful, and the family feared ongoing relationships that might expose them to reprisals.

José's relatives also established distance, without any apparent motives. Soon Jorge's family, which had been significantly involved socially, became isolated—at a time when they were in most need of emotional support. After the kidnapping, a number of changes in family relationships emerged that finally led to consultation with our group.

Jorge was transformed into the awaited one and thus remained "present." His character became progressively idealized. José lost his valued role of productive father, family provider, and protector of his children: his status changed to that of a child, he was now dependent on Marta, and he became progressively more powerless as she became more involved with activities outside the home. The members of the couple were no longer equals.

The family reorganized around Marta. The other family members struggled for her attention. Conflicts between Marta and José emerged in Estela and Guillermo to various degrees and with different levels of awareness on their part. Estela apparently had accepted for many years, without conflict, the departure of her mother from the home, despite the fact that Estela had been an overprotected child as the youngest and only daughter in a rather conventional family. Estela experienced an intense sense of blame toward her mother, linked to her feelings of abandonment. These pre-oedipal issues were intensified by the abrupt modification in family roles within the system. Estela believed that she had no right to raise complaints against her mother, and consciously she supported the role that her mother had assumed. On the other hand, she resented her father's difficulty in maintaining paternal functions and his dependence on her mother.

Marta and José's fear regarding the future of their two other children brought about conflicting situations. Estela was not allowed to develop autonomy during her childhood and adolescence because this involved risks that might lead to dangerous situations. This prohibition applied not only to political beliefs and involvement but also to normal activities related to appropriate developmental tasks, such as traveling alone at night or being away from the house to study. She was forced to maintain an infantile, dependent link to her parents, as well as a devalued role because of the idealization of the disappeared brother. Because of the disappearance, normal feelings of rivalry and jealousy for the parents' love did not emerge. In this family with clear generational boundaries, socially appropriate sexual proscriptions, and clear differentiation between the different selves, a regressive move occurred that reinforced primary processes. This turned the mother into the only provider, disrupted the marital alliance (one result being an almost complete end of sexual intimacy), and disrupted the children's development of self-esteem and independence.

José came to grips with the reality of Argentina's dictatorship and assumed a grandiose responsibility for the destiny of his child. The acceptance of that powerful influence also contributed to his narcissistic collapse. The attitude of his family of origin and the attitudes of his own children and of some of his neighbors reinforced his destructive feelings of guilt. This later led to mutual accusations and blaming within the family. José went on to be imprisoned in his own home, and Marta took over both parental roles. Guillermo and Estela became fixed in their roles as young children. The traumatic effects of terror, and the alienating role models presented by those in power, forced the children to remain dependent well beyond the period appropriate to their life cycles. Although this extension of dependence served to protect the children from real political dangers, it could also be rationalized in a defensive way by Marta, who faced the anguish of accepting the children's becoming independent; Marta thereby postponed her own growth.

Oscar

Silvia, a teacher, and Oscar, an electrical technician, came from different provinces. They were married in Buenos Aires in 1970. Both were politically militant and maintained a cordial relationship with their families of origin. They had two children: Laura, born in 1974, and Daniel, born in June 1976. In December 1976, Oscar was kidnapped on his way to work. Their house was broken into the next day while Laura was at day care and Silvia, with Daniel, was searching for Oscar. When Silvia returned home, she found the door to the apartment damaged and the interior in complete shambles. The television set, stereo, and some other possessions were missing. Terrified, she moved with her children to a friend's house. A few days later, her friends went to her apartment to retrieve her personal belongings and found it practically empty; no furniture, clothes, or dishes were there. Silvia could no longer return to her home. Sometime later, she sold the apartment and, with her family's help, moved to another apartment with her children.

She was unable to obtain any information about her husband's whereabouts. She knew that an uncle of Oscar's and the uncle's wife and brother-in-law had been kidnapped earlier. One of them was released shortly thereafter. He said that he had been tortured and had been repeatedly questioned about several individuals, including Oscar.

Silvia took significant steps to try to locate Oscar and actively participated in meetings (organized by other families) about kidnappings and disappearances. She learned details about her husband's kidnapping 2 years later, by accident; somebody who subsequently joined the human rights movement had witnessed the kidnapping and denounced it before a group of human rights activists. As he was being kidnapped, Oscar had yelled out his name repeatedly, as was the custom in such situations.

Silvia continued to work as a teacher and reorganized her life with her children. She was afraid to discuss the situation with her friends at work, but she maintained an excellent and effective bond with them. She experienced the need to share her anguish but at the same time feared she would lose her job if she revealed that she was the wife of one of the disappeared. The conflict presented itself as a dilemma: she needed support, but she could not speak. Shortly thereafter, she developed a severe phobic syndrome regarding work, and finally she had to stop working.

In spite of her ideological agreement with her husband, during this period she was flooded with hostile feelings toward him for having led her to live in that situation. She blamed him for having disappeared and made accusations never made previously. She felt alone and abandoned by him and at the mercy of a hostile world. She was often extremely aggressive toward her friends, accusing them of not understanding her; at other times she reproached herself for her negative feelings toward those who loved her.

Oscar's family members, who had disapproved of his militancy, distanced themselves from Silvia and did not provide her with any economic assistance, which increased her feelings of hostility and abandonment.

During this period, Silvia found herself torn. She participated in the antidictatorship resistance and protest movement, tolerating the realistic fears of retribution for her activism. However, at a more private level, she identified with changes by the dictatorship that were conducive to guilt and silence. She experienced significant psychological trauma, loss of self-esteem, diminished capacity for adaptation to reality, and neurotic symptoms.

Pressured by the inability to provide for her children and feeling defenseless, Silvia decided to return to her city of origin and resume work. She experienced this decision as a loss of independence and as a personal failure. In her hometown, she continued to have difficulties in resolving emotional and work-related problems, and she developed an infantile dependence on her parents and siblings. She had difficulty forming new relationships, in spite of the fact that she had always been very sociable. She found it difficult to feel stable and rewarded by her work, although she had a good employment record. During the period directly after Oscar's disappearance, Silvia, like most family members who had relatives among the missing, faced the situation of waiting and looking desperately for any information concerning Oscar's whereabouts. At the same time, she began to think that something unpredictable, unknown until that moment, was occurring. Without information that would allow her to appraise the situation realistically, she changed repeatedly in her beliefs: he had been killed, he was a prisoner in an unknown place, he was a prisoner in a place that she had failed to find because of errors in her search, he would be recognized and appear at any time in a known jail, he would return home at any moment and would not find her because of her move.

Her mothering, however, was adequate. She was protective and warm with her children, kept them simply and clearly informed of the events, and attended to their developmental needs with interest and dedication. In addition, after a number of years, she managed to finish her graduate training, found a good professional job, improved her economic situation, and attained a higher status. With time, Silvia became convinced that Oscar would not return.

She wanted to form a new relationship, but the persistence of the uncertainty regarding her husband's return blocked her conscious decision to continue her love life. She thought that if she were to become involved in another relationship, she would be responsible for abandoning Oscar to his destiny. Because bereavement was difficult to process socially in that context, Silvia decided to get divorced. Several years later she remarried, but she maintained her participation in the human rights movement and did not allow her activism to interfere in her relationship with her new husband, who shared her ideas. When Silvia had previously participated in the movement, she had done so as the wife of Oscar. When she began building her new relationship, conflict emerged regarding whether her political friends should know about her remarriage. She feared their censure, in spite of the fact that it was they who had encouraged her to enter into a new relationship. Later on, she disclosed the marriage and subsequently began to experience conflict with her husband. She developed intense feelings of guilt, sexual inhibitions, and irrational fears of the consequences that might result if Oscar returned and found she was married to someone else, although she had never had difficulty in conceptually accepting divorce and the development of new relationships.

Silvia's son Daniel could not comprehend the logic of his father's disappearance and reproached his mother for not looking for him hard enough, repeatedly stating that he would "take care" of finding his father when he grew up. Silvia accepted his accusations as true, thereby reinforcing her self-blame for the abandonment of the disappeared husband. At a conscious level, she considered her activities in the human rights movement not to be incompatible with her new personal situation. She maintained a good relationship with her new husband, who was well accepted by her children.

Silvia underwent two courses of psychotherapy, the first beginning a few months after Oscar's disappearance. More than a year after his disappearance, Silvia said in her therapy that there was no exit: "It is unbearable to think that he may not return, but if he returns in 10 years, for example, who will be returning, and who will I be? We will be two strangers who may not recognize each other." Sometime after moving to her city of origin, she began a second treatment, this time motivated by her wish to form a new relationship. She was also concerned about her periods of decompensation, during which she was flooded with melancholic feelings. She became particularly frightened when she developed alcohol addiction during one of her relapses. During the first period in her therapy, support was of the utmost importance. During the times of uncertainty, she needed someone who could listen, in a nonjudgmental way, to her express her feelings of hostility and hate. Often the therapist had to function as an auxiliary ego to help her resolve concrete issues. The extended family was too preoccupied, collectively processing the significance of the status of their relative (and the link to the disappeared).

Our approach was to support the patient as she was dealing with the lack of definition of her husband's existential status (i.e., existing vs. not existing). Therapeutic interventions helped her separate from the dictatorship's induction of guilt; she was assuming these models as her own instead of understanding her own ambivalent feelings toward her husband and the conflicts previously experienced with him. She was alternatively blaming herself or blaming Oscar for the situation that had victimized both. Her frequent fear of being discovered as the wife of one of the disappeared could be understood at different levels that were mutually reinforcing. It had intimate implications, linked to her personal history, as well as social and environmental connotations, arising from religious convictions (particularly with regard to the concept of sin) acquired during adolescence. That fear was also linked to her identification as a transgressor-sinner, one who was guilty of political militancy and who was the victim of dictatorial repression. These aspects of Silvia's behavior, feelings, and ideas contrasted with her participation in movements of resistance against the dictatorship and with her own general understanding of the attempts at ideological entrapment by the dictatorship.

Therapy also assisted her in reducing the alienating effects of the dominant values of society. This was achieved by reducing reliance on dissociative mechanisms. She was better able to maintain her interpersonal links, accept the affective/positive attachments of those around her, and reduce the intensity of their negative reactions. Her phobic symptoms also diminished, enhancing her ability to deal effectively with reality.

Psychotherapeutic Issues

What is unique in the psychotherapeutic treatment of relatives of the disappeared and victims of political repression in general?

We can elaborate on different modalities of therapy, applicable during different periods depending on the magnitude of the trauma, but the principal concept has to do with the need to analyze the impact of so-called social discourse and its effect on professional practice itself. We understand the phrase *dominant social discourse* to mean the conglomerate of ideas and interpretations about a given situation produced and spread by those in power. This social discourse intervenes as an intrinsic factor in the psychological processing of a traumatic situation.

Frequently, for example, feelings of guilt emerge during the process of bereavement. Our usual interpretation is that the intensity of these feelings relates to the degree of ambivalence present in the relationship: the greater the hostility, the greater the guilt. If guilt feelings now emerge intensely in a traumatic situation that is sociopolitical in origin, and the dominant discourse tends through specific propaganda campaigns to blame parents for the fate of their children, the dynamics of the psychosocial situation change. To interpret feelings of guilt as emanating only from the ambivalent nature of the relationship, or from the personality structure of the individuals, represents a marked limitation in understanding the process. Such an interpretation cannot account for the frequency and consistency of the phenomenon and leads to the intensification of guilt feelings in the patients, resulting in a more difficult process and resolution of the dramatic events.

Neutrality

Our therapeutic stance may conflict with that in traditional psychoanalysis, particularly with regard to the concept of therapeutic neutrality. If the therapist is to be only a screen for the patient's projections, or if his or her own character must be subdued in order to permit the patient's unconscious from being unduly directed, the inclusion of the analysis of social or political aspects of life in therapy would be a breaking of this desired neutrality. We believe that neutrality does not exist in therapy. The therapist's personal decisions emerge in the interpretations or are evident elsewhere: in the style of clothing worn or in the decorations in the office. A neutral stance, furthermore, can contribute to unawareness or its neutralization regarding the influence of social discourse on psychological life. This would perpetuate the socially sanctioned silencing of events, a course much desired by the dictatorship.

A particularly complex problem is that of assuming the disappeared to be dead. During the first years of the dictatorship, family members were led to declare that the disappeared were dead. During this period, some therapists also arrived at similar conclusions due in part to the dominant social discourse and in part to attempts at decreasing the fragmenting effects produced by the ambiguity of the disappearance.

At the same time, any question of responsibility for the deaths was suppressed. In truth, we as therapists knew as little about the fate of the disappeared as did the rest of the population. But soon it became evident to us that the dictatorship would not take charge of elucidating the fate of the disappeared, and the family members had to assume this role.

The relatives also thought they were "killing" the disappeared or abandoning them to their fate. If, in some fashion, this idea was suggested by the therapist, it led to the abrupt termination of treatment or to an increase in feelings of alienation from and lack of understanding of the social milieu. Some relatives learned from witnesses years later that the family member had remained alive for a long time after the family had discontinued the search on the assumption that the family member was dead.

On the other hand, the conviction that the disappeared was still alive could become in some cases an irrational belief, supported by questionable information or by dream content. Our position as therapists was to support the patient, analyze the social process and the different views and options emerging from this analysis, and facilitate the processing experienced by those involved. This involved interpretation of the beliefs in dreams or in clairvoyance, beliefs based on the person's own wish that the disappeared were still alive. This work took place within the previously defined frame of reference, in which the status of the disappeared was denied or negated. This in turn interfered with the process of grief.

The majority of those affected, many led by their own analysis of the facts, arrived over time at the unavoidable conclusion that no persons who had been kidnapped remained alive. When the constitutional government was reinstated, it became possible to share extensive testimony about the facts, which were increasingly becoming public knowledge.

Therapeutic Approaches

If we consider the first years of kidnappings and illegal detentions, we have no doubt that the approach of choice is group therapy, to take place within the settings in which those affected met for exchange of information and the like.

Actually, supportive interventions for those affected by political repression began outside mental health institutions and state hospitals. This was primarily because terror and social silence made those affected fearful of going to official institutions, of telling strangers what was happening to them, or of having political information included in their clinical histories. Another factor of no less importance was the basic need to trust the therapist. Trust is essential in any therapeutic relationship. In situations such as those described, the affected people may expect, as a requirement of trust, to understand the therapist's own stance. The need for trust, then, appears to preclude neutrality.

Conflicts regarding trust led to the emergence of untenable cases, such as the case of a disappeared person's mother who, at 60 years of age, developed psychosis immediately after the kidnapping of her son. She required hospitalization, which was arranged through social service agencies. However, by family consensus, the attending psychiatrist and psychologist were not advised of the essential fact of her son's kidnapping.

Another example is that of a disappeared person's brother who decided to consult the hospital service for marital conflict that he considered totally unrelated to what had occurred to his brother. However, in giving the routine data about his family of origin, he developed persecutory beliefs and decided to terminate the consultation.

For relatives of the disappeared, group therapy is the therapy of choice in the early stages of therapy. The reasons for this are as follows:

- Group therapy respects the model that arose spontaneously in many relatives of the disappeared, that of coming together not only to search for their children but to socialize and process their suffering.
- Because of the nature of group therapy, family members in group therapy do not have to consider themselves to be ill or to be suffering from any type of mental illness as the result of being a victim of political repression. This is especially important for relatives who, in searching for their children, have been repeatedly called "crazy" by the military government and who face denial of the existence of the disappeared.
- Group therapy allows for a better processing of the shared

aspects of the situation, particularly the social discourse and the dominant social representations in the personal suffering produced by the trauma.

- Group therapy helps diminish participants' feeling of isolation.
- If, as in the case of parents of the disappeared, the situation represents an irreparable loss under extreme traumatic conditions, therapeutic interventions at the time of the events facilitate the psychological processing of the situation. The interventions serve as preventive measures against the development of more severe psychological disturbances. In other words, they prevent the emergence of a psychological catastrophe from a social catastrophe.

Individual therapy and family therapy were initially provided when the level of grief was unbearable or when severe depressive episodes emerged. We consider this the therapy of choice in the treatment of middle- and long-term effects. We believe that therapy groups for those affected can reinforce aspects of personal identity attached to the traumatic situation. In addition, the middle- and long-term effects can be more crystallized and may influence the social and affective lives of these people in a much more complex manner; therefore, they may require prolonged psychotherapeutic interventions.

Group Therapy

Our experience with groups began during the years of the military dictatorship, when silence, the attempt at social denial of the existence of the disappeared, was predominant in Argentinian society. There was a need for settings that would allow families to process the subjective traumatic impact that this situation created.

Our team believed there was a manifest request to hold "chats" about themes related to the personal and family processing of patients' experiences. We observed that spontaneous gatherings emerged in the midst of the various tasks performed during searches for missing children. There was an exchange, a more informal and intimate dialogue about personal problems linked to the traumatic situation. In other words, groups were organized so that people could reflect and discuss the themes that changed their lives.

Open groups were formed (attendance was not mandatory) and co-ordinated by one or two professionals from our practice. The number of participants was not limited and has ranged between 15 and 80 people. The group session lasts between 2 and 3 hours. It is necessary to regulate the frequency of these sessions—to prevent them from functioning as inadequate substitutes for other institutional activities requiring a different format and, on the other hand, to prevent the groups' sliding imperceptibly toward becoming sessions of classic therapeutic groups.

In group sessions, all topics that spontaneously arose have been discussed. These topics have varied depending on the various situations developing.

Problems discussed have included such problems as the handling of information about the children of the disappeared, the effect produced by uncertainty, the phenomenon of segregation of the family groups during the period of silence, the changes produced in the role structure of families with the disappearance of one or more members, the management of hostility, and the implications of the assumption that the disappeared person is dead. During the constitutional period, the following themes were prominent: themes linked to the public knowledge of facts about the repression, particularly those facts regarding the living conditions and torture of the detained and disappeared; themes linked to the feelings that developed during exhumations; themes linked to the feelings of guilt and shame in those who did not participate in community events; and themes linked to the interpersonal relationships in the institution. The discussion of these themes was never general but stemmed from the exchange of personal experiences from the group participants. In every group meeting, one or two mothers, often new members of the group, narrated the chronological events of the kidnapping of their child, their first moment of search, and what they felt at that moment and subsequently. A circular dynamic emerged in these groups. When an attempt to monopolize the group occurred, members of the group generally redirected the focus; the group coordinators rarely needed to intervene.

Information flowed, catharsis occurred, members empathized and shared, and different operational models and affective responses were compared.

This group therapy showed that there were needs for participants to provide testimony and to have a shared space for the emergence of the original traumatic situation. There was also a need to record participants' histories, a need that was linked to the personal desire for detailed knowledge of the destiny of each disappeared person,. This need existed because the group members had not been allowed to communicate the true history in a social group.

Group Leader Interventions

As group leaders, we attempt to demonstrate maximum respect and stimulate communication. We avoid monopolizing the attention of group members; on the contrary, we favor all processes of mutual recognition, recognition of differences and similarities, and the capacity to understand and be understood by other group members. Some interventions by leaders are linked to the clarification of complex events. Others begin with issues proposed by members of the group—different repertoires of possible solutions to a similar problem. When necessary, we make individual interpretations, but in general we tend to analyze attitudes and experiences. This may enrich the vision of each of the members of the group toward similar problems.

When the level of idealized demands placed on the coordinator becomes an obstacle to the exchange, we intervene to minimize it. We avoid assuming the role of judge, which could lead to classification of behavior as good or bad, appropriate or inappropriate.

We also establish links between observed affects and the conscious or unconscious ideas on which they are based, verbalize experiences, and associate different situations linked to each other through displacement factors. We expressly avoid transference interpretations, monopolizing interventions (too much talk by the leader), or personal conflicts extraneous to the common problems, even if these are evident to the group.

Observed Effects of Therapy

We have observed direct favorable effects, recognized by the participants themselves, such as decreased guilt. The traumatic situation and the psychological campaign by the dictatorship were of such magnitude that they produced guilt feelings in family members, intensifying bereavement.

These feelings of guilt arose from old conflicts in which ambivalence toward the disappeared played a role, generating a cause-and-effect phenomenon that fosters guilt (e.g., the fantasy that feeling hostility toward the victim may have played some role in the kidnapping). The discussion of these themes in a group setting made evident, through the interchange of subjective experiences, how convictions of guilt held throughout the years by some group members clashed with feelings of guilt in others, who were supported by exactly the opposite beliefs.

Other favorable effects have included a decrease in distress and increased stress tolerance. Catharsis, verbal exchange, and the multiple phenomena discussed in relationship to the group process impinge on these aspects. There were discriminating and clarifying effects, in particular the rupture of certain types of massive or condensed identifications (e.g., there developed an ability to recognize and tolerate the different effects in the children and in the mother of the disappeared induced by the disappearance). In this way, the internal logic that determines different behaviors was able to be understood.

Finally, maintenance and reinforcement of self-esteem through support and reorientation were assisted by the reality principle and comprehension of problems between the ego and the ego ideal. Self-esteem was also reinforced when family and social group activities were validated.

Unsystematized Psychological Interventions

We designate as unsystematized psychological interventions certain clinically important activities that facilitate bonding with family members of the disappeared. Family members themselves have recognized these as therapeutic and have pointed out their effectiveness to us. These interventions emerged with the permanent and informal insertion of the members of the professional team into the natural group and institution.

As we proposed, the family members of the disappeared developed spontaneous group activities, which created a place for psychological support in the difficult circumstances. Everyday issues were shared, including different tasks to be solved, as well as domestic concepts and more general political concerns. In this way, links allowing the emergence and discussion of various personal, family, and even institutional problems were generated. Our presence within these activities demanded spontaneous reactions beyond our technically therapeutic roles.

Interventions in these cases were aimed at facilitating a permissive institutional dynamic, in which different positions toward the same problem were held by members of the group. Group members were never coerced or attacked for favoring points of views differing from those of the majority or of the leaders of the group.

Because of prejudice and lack of previous information about psychological therapies, many individuals were unlikely to accept psychological treatment with commitment. However, because of the trust and closeness that developed with the professional group, members accepted more informal individual sessions, which made it possible for them to process situations of conflict and moments of crisis, to accept the roles of others, or to make some other defenses more flexible. These informal sessions emerged from the group's sense of confidence produced by the members' direct acquaintance and familiarity with us in the meetings of the natural group. This arrangement constituted a therapeutic space that could be open or closed according to the needs that arose, not necessarily with temporal continuity.

Another situation that emerged frequently resulted from the aging of some of the family members, a process accompanied by organic disorders with subsequent distress and feelings of abandonment. These feelings were intensified by the failure of the state and social assistance agencies to provide adequate medical care or even explain the prognosis of the ailments.

Accompanying individuals to various appointments and providing follow-up notes to colleagues in other specialties resulted in clarifying discussions about diagnosis, treatment, and prognosis. This reduced anxiety not only for the person affected but for the entire group. It also improved understanding of the pathology, whether organic, hypochondriacal, or psychosomatic.

It was also useful to develop a network of medical colleagues who were involved in the defense of human rights, so that specialized services could be provided. In addition to permitting concrete clinical problems to be resolved, this network provided for the patients the containment and protection necessitated by the patients' feelings of abandonment and helplessness.

Assisting families of the disappeared and alleviating their suffering are duties of physicians. This work involves the interplay of social commitment and professional function.

References

Freud S: Mourning and melancholia (1917), in Standard Edition of the Complete Psychological Works of Sigmund Freud, Vol 14. Translated and edited by Strachey J. London, Hogarth Press, 1959, pp 237–258

Freud S: Preface to Psychoanalysis and War Neuroses (1919), in Standard Edition of the Complete Psychological Works of Sigmund Freud, Vol 17. Translated and edited by Strachey J. London, Hogarth Press, 1959, pp 205–215

Freud S: Inhibitions, symptoms, and anxiety (1926), in Standard Edition of the Complete Psychological Works of Sigmund Freud, Vol 20. Translated and edited by Strachey J. London, Hogarth Press, 1959, pp 77–174

Kordon D, Edelman L: Psychological Effects of Political Repression. Buenos Aires, Sudamerica/Planeta, 1986

Laplanche J, Pontalis JB: Diccionario de psicoanàlisis, 1st Edition. Santiago, Chile, Empressa Editora Nacional Quimantu Lemetado, 1972

CHAPTER 13

Caring for
Survivors of Torture
Beyond the Clinic

Aurora A. Parong, M.D.

People enter the health profession for a host of reasons. For those who choose to care for survivors of torture, the reasons go beyond the intellectual, scientific, and pecuniary. Pledging to consecrate one's life to the service of humanity is, perhaps, never more highly expressed than in caring for torture survivors, especially in areas such as the Philippines, where state repression puts the lives of health care professionals at risk.

Filipino physicians and other health care workers engaged in the rehabilitation of survivors of torture debunk the still predominant notion that disease is determined primarily by biological factors. They adopt the view that physical and chemical laws govern disease mechanisms but must be seen to operate within a social and economic context (Doyal 1979).

Physicians in the Philippines go beyond the clinics and hospitals to assist survivors of torture. They perform various functions, being involved in the provision of medical, physical, surgical, and psychological care, as well as in research and the development of effective methods and approaches for relief and rehabilitation work. Physicians also may work hard to obtain justice for the survivors of torture and may zealously campaign for an end to the unhampered human rights violations in the country.

Philippine Realities

Seventy percent of Filipinos live below the poverty line because land and natural resources of the country have been owned and controlled for centuries by a few, who also wield political power. The Philippine economy has always been subservient to industrialized countries, particularly the United States. This exploitative situation has given rise to armed and unarmed social and political movements. The Philippine government has persistently used repressive measures to quell these movements.

Although the Philippines is a signatory to conventions against torture, torture occurs in the Philippines. The ouster of the late dictator Ferdinand Marcos and the assumption of power by Corazon Aquino in a February 1986 popular uprising did not alter the situation.

Task Force Detainees of the Philippines (TFDP), a human rights monitoring organization, reported the torture of 2,401 persons, or 16% of all persons arrested by the military during the first 3 years (1986–1989) of the Aquino government. Nearly a thousand who were not arrested were physically and mentally assaulted by military personnel (Task Force Detainees of the Philippines 1989).

In a 1987–1990 study by the Balay Rehabilitation Center (BALAY), the Medical Action Group (MAG), and TFDP,[1] the most common methods of torture noted in 62 cases in the Manila metropolitan area were mauling (94%), threats of death or injury to the person or loved ones (58%), assault with a weapon (44%), "water cure" (29%),[2] strangulation (23%), removal of clothing (21%), suffocation (18%), and electric shock (16%).

---

[1]"Incidents of Torture in the Nations Capital Region," a report submitted to Mr. Kojima, the United Nations' Committee on Human Rights Special Rapporteur on Torture, when he visited the Philippines in 1990.

[2]"Water cure" can be performed in any of the following ways: by submerging the head in water to induce near suffocation; by pouring pepper-laced water into the nose and mouth; by immersing the head in a toilet bowl containing urine and feces; or by pouring water into the nose while the back is kept against the floor.

A post-Marcos phenomenon of mass torture has likewise surfaced. The victims are terrorized by indiscriminate bombings of their communities, the burning and strafing of their houses, and the "salvaging"[3] of their relatives. In the government's effort to drive off so-called state enemies, communities are subjected to prolonged military operations and are isolated and denied access to food and medicines. The victims are called *internal refugees.*[4]

From 1987 to September 1989, a total of 85,022 displaced families (485,832 persons) were reported by the Department of Social Welfare and Development (Tanada 1990). In 1990, there were 22,561 families displaced from their homes as a result of relentless military operations. These are alarming numbers, and there are many unreported cases of internal refugees. With a policy of "total war"[5] against dissidents still very much in place, the figures are likely to increase.

Essential Considerations

Filipino health care professionals work within a biopsychosocial framework in assisting survivors of torture. They also consider and confront the socioeconomic and political order, which is at the heart of the occurrence of torture. A holistic approach is achieved by taking into account all of the following factors: 1) culture and subculture, 2) family and community, 3) the economic situation, and 4) the political situation.

---

[3]*Salvaging,* a term that was commonly used during the Marcos dictatorship, means summary execution or extrajudicial execution.

[4]"Report of International Fact-Finding Mission on Internal Refugees." Mission was conducted in the Philippines October 23–November 1, 1989, by a team with members from Australia, Canada, Germany, Netherlands and Switzerland.

[5]The Total War Policy against the insurgents was instituted by President Corazon Aquino after the collapse of the peace talks between the government and the National Democratic Front, the underground armed opposition. The Total War Policy includes "population control," which is defined by the Ecumenical Movement for Justice and Peace as "military tactics to separate the masses from the insurgents taken from the premise that the insurgency is largely dependent on a supportive populace . . . the masses are the water, the insurgents are the fish . . . military drains the water by forcing village folks to evacuate or flee to 'safer grounds,' which is usually a place in the urban community, near a military detachment, which can be easily sealed off or monitored."

Culture and Subculture

Knowledge of culture is most important in the care of survivors of torture because cultural differences have implications in the assessment of mental health, in the interpretation of a respondent's behavior or response, and in the treatment or rehabilitation technique (Hauff 1992).

However, Bartolome (1990), a Filipino sociologist, warned of the uncritical application of observed values, traits, and virtues across all strata in a highly stratified society like the Philippines.

Long years of colonization have produced the prevailing subservient culture and consciousness among Filipinos, that is, meekness and silence in the face of oppression and exploitation, as well as superior regard for foreign ideas and goods. Filipinos are observed to be family- and small-group-oriented, as well as paternalistic.

But many contrasting values and ideals have been noted that may be due to distinctions between urban and rural settings and to influences of social class (Marcelino 1990). There have likewise evolved a counter-culture and counterconsciousness associated with the movements for social change in the Philippines. These factors were developed during the long years of colonization and during the Marcos dictatorship.

Thus, a mixture of subcultures, some conflicting, is highly manifest in Philippine society. Some groups maintain the status quo. However, Filipinos who are actively working for radical changes in the country— and who, in most cases, are the victims of torture—advocate and live in an almost entirely different culture. This culture includes group consciousness, high regard for collective responsibilities and efforts, and the ability to confront hardships and difficulties because of strong commitments to social reform.

When internal refugees ascribe to this counterculture, most often they are able to organize themselves and develop activities to keep their morale high and to alleviate their situations. Their responses include documenting their conditions, constructing security measures, participating in the distribution of relief goods, and building temporary shelters.

Family and Community

Strained interpersonal relationships, changes in roles and expectations, differences in political perspectives, and communal sharing of resources are important variables to consider when attempting to understand not only the survivors, but also their families and communities. Most of the time, the social and economic situations of the survivors and their families are radically restructured, and these situations often lead to prolonged, repeated, and severe stress.

The typically Asian extended family system in the Philippines is usually the main support network that survives after the social and economic dislocation of the nuclear family. In these situations, families who reaffirm or, at the very least, understand the political choices of the survivors are much more helpful therapeutically.

Communities, too, play a significant role in the rehabilitation of individual survivors of torture. Especially in rural areas, members of the community are treated in many ways like members of the family. Extended families are usually found in the same contiguous area or community. In the case of internal refugees, the absence of communities to which one can return further aggravates feelings of helplessness and despair. But the extended family's home sometimes serves as a sanctuary for survivors who were displaced because of massive and prolonged military operations.

Economic Situation

Most torture survivors come from the marginalized sectors of Philippine society. They are generally workers, peasants, and members of the lower middle class.

In a 1986 survey conducted by an organization of former detainees,[6] 42% of 100 subjects considered economics to be a cause of their difficulties after release from detention. At the Children's Rehabilitation Center (CRC), an institution that renders services to children who are victims of human rights violations, 44% of patients between 1985 and 1988 had financial and economic problems (Marcelino 1989). On the other hand, internal refugees forced from their farmlands and deprived of other sources of livelihood faced hunger and disease.

---

[6]Samahan ng mga Ex-Detainees Laban sa Detensyon at Para sa Amnestiya (SELDA), Socio-Economic Survey of Ex-Political Detainees in Four Areas of the Philippines, Manila, The Philippines, 1986.

Families of torture survivors under detention suffer economic dislocation, especially if the detainees are the main breadwinners. Family
members are usually fully occupied with their own survival and neglect
seeking assistance for the survivors of torture. Experience has shown that
providing direct material and economic aid to survivors and their families
contributes immensely to overall adjustment.

Political Situation

The government's counterinsurgency campaign remains the major cause
of torture and other forms of human rights violations.[7] At the same time,
it constitutes the single largest obstacle to the rehabilitation of torture survivors. Threats to life and security are realities confronting the survivors
of torture, as well as health care professionals. It is not uncommon for
political prisoners to suffer repeated traumatic experiences during detention. Former detainees continue to suffer from stress because of the high
possibility of recapture or reprisals from the agents of the state who were
responsible for their torture. In 1988, two detainees complained of repeated torture experiences in prison, experiences that were still occurring
even after the Supreme Court had been informed about the torture perpetrated by the detainees' captors.[8] In a 1986 survey of 100 former detainees
in four areas of the Philippines,[9] 49 detainees responded that concerns
regarding security were a cause of their difficulties in adjusting to life after
imprisonment.

It is difficult to start life anew amid conditions of repression in the

---

[7] A report by the Philippine Senate Committee on Justice and Human Rights in 1990
(Tanada 1990) concluded that "the total approach strategy is considered a major factor
contributing to the continuing human rights violations. . . . Because of the total war policy, the accommodation of democratic dissent and respect for human rights is made more
difficult."

[8] MAG files, 1988. The survivors of torture were released from detention, and the cases
filed against them were dismissed because of insufficient evidence. The government did
not take action against the perpetrators of the torture.

[9] Samahan ng mga Ex-Detainees Laban sa Detensyon at Para sa Amnestiya (SELDA), Socio-
Economic Survey of Ex-Political Detainees in Four Areas of the Philippines, Manila, The
Philippines, 1986.

country. Internal refugees, who may be able to cope easily with initial traumatic experiences, reach their limits when subjected to prolonged traumatic situations. When refugees are desperate, rendering assistance to them becomes even more complex and difficult. For example, in October 1991 an elderly woman from Marag Valley[10] asked for poison to end her life. Four of her grandchildren, after being displaced because of massive military operations, had died from measles complicated by bronchopneumonia. Two other relatives had been summarily executed by the military, and another relative had been raped several times. The woman had accepted the first deaths in the family courageously, but the subsequent ones, along with the illnesses, the continued bombings, and the military harassments, combined to take a toll on her (Canila 1991).

Providing assistance to internal refugees in the Philippines proves very difficult given the atmosphere of political strife. Epidemics and deaths in evacuation centers have occurred despite the provision of services by government health agencies, which have often been a liability rather than an asset. The military or paramilitary units on guard have prevented refugees from seeking the assistance of nongovernmental organizations.

Health care professionals assisting torture survivors are not exempt from military abuses. Health care teams have been subjected to various kinds of harassments, including threats to life, interrogations, and actual detention while visiting political prisoners (Medical Action Group, unpublished letter and affidavits, November 1990).[11] There have been incidents in which health care personnel, Filipinos, and foreigners were

---

[10]Marag Valley, in the northern Philippines, has lush forests and rich reserves of gold and other minerals. Loggers and miners, who benefited from the rich resources of the valley, were driven out by the people and by the New People's Army and the National Democratic Front. They retaliated in cooperation with the military and their private armies. In 1985, Marag and neighboring towns were declared no-man's-land. Food suupply blockage, media blockage, and restriction of movement of the people were imposed, and massive military operations were relentlessly conducted. More than 100 internal refugee children died from measles and bronchopneumonia in 1991.

[11]November 19, 1990, letter from the Medical Action Group to the Commission on Human Rights regarding harassment of a MAG health care team by police authorities at the Navotas Municipal Jail on November 14, 1990, and November 1990 affidavits of members of the health care team.

intimidated and detained by military and paramilitary groups and were therefore prevented from conducting medical missions in refugee areas (Medical Action Group 1987, 1988, 1990).

Rehabilitation of torture survivors is very difficult in the face of continuing repression. Health care workers assisting them must recognize this reality.

Roles of Psychiatrists and Other Physicians

Various roles, within and outside the confines of the clinics, are filled by psychiatrists and other physicians who care for survivors of torture in the Philippines.

Treatment Providers

At the MAG outpatient clinic in 1990, 52 of 458 persons—torture survivors and their relatives—were given psychological assistance, and most of these persons were treated medically (Medical Action Group 1990). Some survivors have been treated for direct physical effects of torture. However, many torture survivors have been held incommunicado for several days so that, when the primary care physician or psychiatrist finally sees them, the physical signs of torture have usually healed.

Child victims of violence seen at the CRC have been treated for bruises, scratches, lacerations, broken arms or legs, and ruptured eardrums (Marcelino 1992). Common medical problems caused or aggravated by detention or displacement include tuberculosis, pneumonia, upper respiratory infections, diarrhea, and measles. Among internal refugees, diarrhea and measles complicated by bronchopneumonia have taken the lives of more than 100 children in various parts of the country.

Treatment of the survivor's medical problems invariably affects his or her psychological condition. Physical therapy, medicines, and surgical procedures all help the survivor regain trust in other people—trust that may have been lost because of the torture experience.

Somatization, or the expression of emotional distress in the form of bodily symptoms, is a common occurrence among Filipinos. Bodily pains, headache, or malaise may be the presenting complaints of survivors who have feelings of guilt and worthlessness (Lopez 1989). Care should be taken to distinguish the psychosomatic problems from documented physical problems.

Real and actual threats to the life and security of the survivors need to be distinguished from mere illusions and delusions of persecution if torture survivors are to be assisted effectively. Failure to make these distinctions can jeopardize survivors' lives or result in the provision of inappropriate interventions.

For torture survivors with psychological problems, individual counseling and psychotherapy, group therapy, and/or intrafamily and interfamily counseling should be provided. For adults, stress reduction therapy and occupational therapy may be helpful. For children, play activities should be scheduled.

In a therapeutic relationship, trust is essential. Trust and an effective therapeutic relationship are facilitated when the health care provider knows and understands the sociopolitical context under which torture occurs. The provider must understand—if not accept, share, or validate—the political views of the survivor.

To provide assistance effectively, physicians work with other professionals, including psychologists, dentists, nurses, and social workers. They also coordinate and collaborate with groups who give legal aid, economic assistance, and other support.

In the Philippines, three institutions provide the majority of health services to survivors of torture. The CRC renders primarily psychological assistance to child victims of torture and human rights abuse. MAG provides medical and psychological assistance to survivors of torture, be they detainees, former detainees, or internal refugees. BALAY meets former detainees' medical and psychological needs. These centers usually employ physicians of various specialties, psychologists, nurses, and social workers. Services are provided not only in the centers, but also in the communities, evacuation centers, detention centers, and even survivors' homes.

Developers of Effective Methods and Approaches

Most of the literature on relief and rehabilitation work among torture survivors refers to experiences in developed countries and among refugees in exile. There is a dearth of reports on experiences in developing countries in which repression continues.

In the Philippines, most of the activities of the rehabilitation programs remain action oriented and generally short term. This is because of the increasing number of survivors seeking assistance and the few available health care workers.

Health care professionals, including psychiatrists and other physicians, psychologists, and social workers, especially from the CRC, MAG, BALAY, Akademya ng Sikolohiyang Pilipino (Philippine Psychology Research and Training House), and the University of the Philippines, have been able to conduct a modest amount of research in conjunction with their work. Studies have characterized the patient population in terms of the common physical and psychological problems, complaints, patterns of torture, and the various responses of both child and adult survivors of torture. Efforts have been made to determine the essential factors (individual, social, economic, and political) affecting the traumatic experience and the response of the patient population. There also have been efforts to determine the efficacy of therapeutic approaches and techniques, particularly selected therapies relevant to certain cultures and populations.

Methodologies used in these studies have been indigenous and participatory. They include *pagtatanong-tanong* (Filipino term meaning *questioning*) and *pakikipagkuwentuhan* (mutual storytelling).[12] The experiences and conditions of the torture survivors have been analyzed from the point of view of the survivors themselves and of their social group. Some of these studies have been presented in various local and international conferences; most remain unpublished at present.

Providers of Mental Health Education and Training

Psychiatrists and other physicians assign importance to strengthening the coping mechanisms of individuals in high-risk groups and to the role of

---

[12]Pagtatanong-tanong and pakikipagkuwentuhan are indigenous research methods promoted by the Akademya ng Sikolohiyang Pilipino. These methods were used by Claudio, Bartolome, and Dalisay in the Pilot Study on Children in Crisis, conducted in 1989, the results of which were presented in the First International Seminar-Workshop on Children in Crisis held in the Philippines.

other direct-service workers in assisting torture survivors.

Education concerning the nature and objectives of torture and the coping mechanisms has been offered to high-risk groups in the Filipino population. High-risk groups include those persons involved in the movement for societal change, members and staff of cause-oriented groups, and residents of communities subject to militarization. Some of these efforts have been conducted by MAG.

The psychologists of the CRC have conducted training for human rights organization workers, who usually are among the first to see torture survivors. This kind of training is to be expanded to include families of torture survivors.

Materials for training and public education have been developed and have evolved. The CRC has produced materials such as *Sikolohiyang Pilipino at Pagbibigay ng Tulong* (Filipino Psychology and Rendering Services), *Ang Katangian ng Isang Biktima* (Characteristics of a Victim), and *Pakikinig at Pagbibigay ng Payo, Batayang Pagsasanay para sa Direct Service Workers* (Listening and Counseling, Basic Training for Direct Service Workers). MAG has also published materials, including *Torture Survivors—What Can We Do for Them?* and *Pagtulong sa Biktima ng Tortyur—Isang Gabay* (Assistance to Victims of Torture—A Guide).

Further work is needed to develop more effective materials for public education and training together with improved approaches for implementation.

Procurers of Justice

Although many may consider obtaining justice for the survivors to be beyond the purview of psychiatrists and other physicians, health care providers in the Philippines participate in this endeavor.

Justice denied is a persistent irritant to the psychological wounds of a torture survivor. Therefore, the importance of working for justice must not and cannot be underrated.

Filipino psychiatrists and other physicians have offered medical, psychological, and forensic documentation of torture to the courts. In 1990, Amnesty International (1990) reported that the harshest punishment for perpetrators of torture in the Philippines was discharge from military service. Under President Aquino's administration, only three military officers received such punishment. However, health care workers in the

Philippines continue such documentation and continue to give testimony in courts in the hope of obtaining justice for the survivors.

A class-action suit filed against Ferdinand Marcos by survivors of torture was concluded in a district court in Hawaii. In January 1995, the case was decided in favor of compensation for the plaintiffs. The prosecution's case rested on the testimony of physicians as well as on the reports of the survivors.

Crusaders for Justice, Peace, and Respect for Human Rights

The prevention of torture is part and parcel of human rights work. Human rights education and advocacy for social justice are vital because although psychological and physical wounds of torture heal, scars remain in the hearts and minds of survivors and the general population. If the society in which survivors live continues to tolerate human rights violations, rehabilitation can never be fully achieved. As violations escalate, the society establishes more rehabilitation programs instead of maximizing efforts and resources for development and improvement of the lives of its people.

Human rights education ensures that the people know their rights and are aware of the means by which rights can be enforced and protected. Human rights advocacy serves to promote and protect such rights.

Working for the protection and promotion of human rights is controversial among health care professionals. Many want to avoid "political" concerns and to concentrate on "health" concerns. This position is advocated by physicians who remain committed to the view that disease is determined purely by biological factors; this perspective is often propagated in medical and other health institutions. Involvement in political issues in a country in which "members of the opposition" often become victims of human rights violations is risky. Moreover, it is not financially rewarding.

For those involved in the care of survivors of torture, to avoid "politics" is to escape from the reality that the problem of torture is not purely a psychological or medical concern. In the context of the Philippines, it is only a symptom of a disintegrating socioeconomic and political order.

A few psychiatrists and other physicians have taken concrete action to strike at the economic and political factors that greatly affect the health and lives of the torture survivors. These professionals have drafted letters of appeal to governments and to international bodies, demanding intervention to alleviate the sufferings of victims of human rights violations. They have written open letters denouncing the torture of political detainees and the harassment of health care professionals. They have initiated appeals for the investigation of cases of human rights abuse and have joined fact-finding missions to document violations and make public these findings.

Some physicians, although theoretically convinced that the economic and political context must be acknowledged in the practice of medicine, have difficulties concretizing their views. Painstaking efforts are necessary to help these individuals reconceptualize their responsibilities as health care providers.

A distinct social, economic, and political context exists in the Philippines that requires a distinct response from psychiatrists, primary care physicians, and other health care professionals. The risks associated with the care of survivors of torture demand a higher commitment from the health profession.

References

Amnesty International: 1990 Report. London, Amnesty International Publications, 1990

Bartolome JM: The pitfalls of Filipino personality, in Indigenous Psychology. Edited by Enriquez V. Quezon City, The Philippines, Akademya ng Sikolohiyang Pilipino, 1990

Canila C: Vilma Alejandro: Where the terror of the total war policy ends up. Progress Notes 5:3–4, 1991

Doyal L, Pennell I: The Political Economy of Health. London, Pluto Press, 1979

Hauff E: Psychosocial work with refugees: a challenge to public health workers, in Health Situation of Refugees and Victims of Organized Violence. Rijswijk, Ministry of Welfare, Health and Cultural Affairs, 1992, pp 105–116

Lopez J: The psychological aspects of torture as seen among Filipino torture victims. Paper presented at the 8th World Congress of Psychiatry, Athens, Greece, October 13–19, 1989

Marcelino E: Psychological help to children victims of political violence. Paper presented at the 5th Asian Workshop on Child and Adolescent Development, Quezon City, The Philippines, February 24, 1989

Marcelino E: Towards understanding the Filipino psychology, in Diversity and Complexity in Feminist Therapy. Edited by Brown L, Root M. New York, Harrington Press, 1990

Marcelino E: Children in crisis: the effects of war on children. Children of the Storm. July 1991–March 1992, 2–3(1–2):25, 1992

Medical Action Group: Cases of Human Rights Violations to Health Professionals and Health Workers: 1987 Survey Report. Manila, The Philippines, Medical Action Group, 1987

Medical Action Group: Cases of Human Rights Violations to Health Professionals and Health Workers: 1988 Survey Report. Manila, The Philippines, Medical Action Group, 1988

Medical Action Group: Cases of Human Rights Violations to Health Professionals and Health Workers: 1989 Survey Report. Manila, The Philippines, Medical Action Group, 1989

Tanada W: Report of the Committee on Justice and Human Rights on the Human Rights Situation in the Philippines. Manila, The Philippines, Committee on Justice and Human Rights, 1990

Task Force Detainees of the Philippines: The Human Rights Record of the Aquino Government. Task Force Detainees of the Philippines, November 29, 1989

CHAPTER 14

Caring for Victims on Site
Bosnian Refugees in Croatia

Suzanne Witterholt, M.D.
James M. Jaranson, M.D., M.A., M.P.H.

Often, the treatment for victims of torture takes place, if it takes place at all, in a country of asylum far from the survivor's native land. Treatment is rarely initiated until months and often years after the torture.

International agencies and the world community respond to crises, such as the violence in the former Yugoslavia, with as much physical support as they can muster. Many physicians, from primary care physicians to surgeons, have a significant role to play in such crises. However, attention to the psychiatric and psychological consequences continues to be delayed until some later date when the confusion and chaos have subsided. Unfortunately, as is known from the treatment of soldiers during wartime, ignoring these considerations early on may make the recovery process more difficult and prolonged (Camp 1993). An analogous situation would be that of a man who breaks his leg while living where he has no access to medical care. The bone may be set haphazardly and heal improperly. Later, when he reaches a hospital, the man will have to have his leg refractured and reset, and he will face a more arduous recovery.

Precedents exist for treating posttraumatic stress symptoms on site. For example, the U.S. military regularly employs psychiatrists and other mental health professionals in war zones. Many of the techniques used to mitigate traumatic reactions could certainly be, and sometimes are, used in refugee camps (Fletcher et al. 1993). In the United States, mental health professionals frequently work at the scenes of disaster, such as areas where there have been floods or tornadoes, to help triage victims with acute reactions while educating and giving support to the victims regarding the nature of posttraumatic stress reactions and their treatment.

People who care for victims of political violence frequently become traumatized themselves as they listen to the horrors described. Posttraumatic stress symptoms can be experienced by these clinicians, even when the clinicians are working in the best of circumstances. The problem is magnified when one must treat survivors in a setting of ongoing violence. Clinicians report changes in their worldview and often find themselves altering their lives to accommodate such changes. For example, we (the authors) have limited the types of movies and plays we see and the books we read because of our growing inability to tolerate displays of violence. This phenomenon of vicarious traumatization can be detrimental to the helpers and ultimately render them unable to give adequate support (McCann and Pearlman 1990).

In contrast to caregivers in countries of final resettlement, those in war zones have little chance for respite. There are usually too few professionals to meet the overwhelming needs, and those professionals who are available often do not attend to their own mental health needs. The need for regular team meetings and debriefing sessions is too often overlooked when groups go into war zones (Loveridge 1993). When rescue teams ignore their own mental health requirements, they cannot be responsive to the mental health needs of the victims.

In this chapter, we describe the situation in Bosnia as it existed in February 1993. We also discuss two intervention approaches by the U.S. Agency for International Development (AID) and the Center for Victims of Torture (CVT) in Minneapolis, Minnesota. These approaches are 1) bringing program directors and health care professionals from the former Yugoslavia to the United States for training and respite and 2) assisting workers in a program in Croatia to intervene quickly with torture victims, using local resources.

The Bosnian Example

In February 1993, one of us (S.W.) had the opportunity to travel to Croatia as a consultant for AID. This particular trip was in response to the horrifying revelations that Serbian forces were killing, torturing, and raping thousands of Bosnians in a campaign of "ethnic cleansing." Whole villages were being rounded up, and all persons in the villages, with men separated from women and children, were forced into concentration camps (World Conference on Human Rights 1993). Media attention was focused on the use of sexual violence as a military tactic. On January 9, 1993, the *New York Times* quoted a report by a European Community investigation in which it was estimated that at least 20,000 Muslim women had been raped by Serbian soldiers (Riding 1993). According to the United Nations High Commissioner for Refugees, by November 1992 five million people had been displaced or had become refugees within the former Yugoslavia as a result of the violence (U.S. Agency for International Development 1993). By the time of the trip, at least one million refugees and displaced persons were staying in Croatia, with the vast majority living in private homes. The situation was complicated by a failing economy and by ethnic tensions in Croatia itself, which were exacerbated by the presence of so many victims of the fighting. Furthermore, the mental health care system, which was primarily a system of state-run hospitals for the chronically mentally ill and which existed in a society in which rape and incest were still not discussed, was hardly prepared for the onslaught of so many highly traumatized people (Anthony et al. 1993; Fletcher et al. 1993).

In the refugee centers visited by the team, mental health services were for the most part not provided (World Conference on Human Rights 1993). The psychological needs of the caregivers were not met (Loveridge 1993). Few if any psychotropic medications were available, and those that were usually were date-expired medications given by United States pharmaceutical companies.

A case in point was the United Nations Transit Center for Bosnians released from concentration camps. Located in the Croatian town of Karlovac, the transit center had been established in October 1992 to facilitate the movement of refugees into areas of asylum. In February 1993, this camp housed approximately 2,000 refugees, most of whom had been victims of torture, as evidenced by their Serbian concentration camp experiences, which included daily beatings, malnourishment, and rape.

Many had been held at the prison camp in Omarska, described by the manager of the transit center as a "killing machine." The refugees experienced the trauma of exile and the stress of uncertainty as they waited for asylum; the camp at Karlovac was only 1 kilometer from the front line and, at the time of the visit, was shelled on a regular basis. The part of the camp housing the majority of the women and children, who numbered 500, had a bomb shelter equipped for only 200 people.

Most of the refugees had symptoms of hypervigilance, increased startle reactions, decreased sleep punctuated with nightmares, and intrusive recollections of the torture alternating with numbing and decreased energy. The Croatian physicians who ran the camp's medical service reported that the most frequent complaints were nightmares, flashbacks, panic, and social withdrawal, often complicated by alcohol abuse resulting in violent behavior. Psychosomatic complaints were also common and increased after a weekend of shelling. None of the physicians were psychiatrists. As might be expected, they expressed frustration at the lack of trained personnel or proper medications for effective treatment of patients suffering from overwhelming psychological distress.

This transit center had approximately 2,000 victims of torture who continued to be traumatized by shelling, overcrowded conditions, and lack of certainty about the future. Much attention was being given to physical ailments such as infectious diseases, whereas mental health problems were left untreated because of a lack of resources. The world community had responded with shipments of much-needed antibiotics and bandages but had disregarded the deep psychological distress that was certain to take a toll on these refugees.

Intervention Strategies

A number of approaches for addressing the psychiatric and psychological needs of victims on site are plausible. First some caveats should be given. The former Yugoslavia is just one example of cases in which organizations from other countries could choose, or have chosen, to intervene. Each example is unique, but some general approaches may apply to different sites. Risks include bringing models of treatment that, although applicable in their original context, do not work on site. There can be a tendency for those from the outside to ignore or minimize the cultural and sociopolitical context and to assume that the model will work universally without modification. Realistically, although those caregivers from elsewhere may have much to offer, it is inappropriate for them to assume they have a better knowledge of the situation than do the caregivers on site.

In addition, there is the risk of poor coordination and duplication of services when many organizations enter a given area of ongoing violence. In the former Yugoslavia, many governmental and nongovernmental organizations have offered mental health services or plan to incorporate them into their existing programs. A few of the governmental organizations are the World Health Organization and the United Nations High Commission for Refugees; the Croatian government has also offered mental health services. Nongovernmental organizations include the American Refugee Committee, the International Rescue Committee, and the International Rehabilitation Council for Torture Victims (Arcel et al. 1995). Efforts have been made to coordinate the activities of the organizations offering help.

The situation in the former Yugoslavia is rapidly changing, and, by the time this book is published, many of the details will undoubtedly have changed. Concerning the program in Croatia, where most are located, there are a number of problems. First of all, there is little history of nongovernmental organizations in the former Yugoslavia, and most of the local organizations are directed by clinicians who have no prior management experience. Second, camps supported by Muslim organizations are difficult for Croatians and other outsiders to enter, although most camps are under the auspices of the Croatian government. Third, it is estimated that more than half of all refugees live illegally outside camps in the former Yugoslavia and are not able to register in the country. Consequently, it is difficult to identify and help them.

Offering services to torture victims on site is one strategy. Another is to intervene in transit camps outside the former Yugoslavia (e.g., Switzerland) and, of course, in the countries of final resettlement (e.g., the United States).

Yet another intervention strategy is to provide health professionals or caregivers with respite, debriefing, and training. This is necessary on site and should be incorporated formally or informally into programs in the former Yugoslavia. However, it is often helpful or even necessary to remove the caregivers from the ongoing violence to safer places. This has been done by the Rehabilitation and Research Centre for Tor-

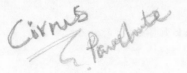

ture Victims in Copenhagen, for example, and by the Centre de Soins de l'AVRE in Paris.

Assisting Local Providers: Projects of the Center for Victims of Torture

CVT has used several of the intervention strategies described in the previous section to help those from the former Yugoslavia. We will discuss two of CVT's projects: 1) a training program at CVT for professionals and paraprofessionals selected from the former Yugoslavia by AID and 2) onsite activities by CVT in the former Yugoslavia. Many organizations besides CVT have conducted similar activities with former Yugoslavians. The two CVT projects outlined here serve as examples of how a relatively small and resource-poor center can help.

First of all, however, a description of the evolution of CVT is called for to elucidate the process that has led CVT to reach out beyond the confines of its geographic location. CVT was established in 1985 and became the first comprehensive, staffed center designed specifically for torture victims. The mandate of CVT is to provide comprehensive treatment to the victims of government-sponsored torture and their families; to conduct research on treatment and rehabilitation models; to provide professional training to other care providers throughout the world; and to contribute to the prevention of torture through public education, public policy initiatives, and cooperative efforts with human rights organizations. Further details of CVT's development and its multidisciplinary treatment model are given by Garcia-Peltoniemi and Jaranson (1989) and Chester (1990).

CVT remains the only comprehensive program of its type in the United States and has provided leadership internationally in the development and provision of comprehensive assessment, treatment, and support services for torture survivors. It is an independent, nonprofit agency staffed by primary care physicians, psychiatrists, nurses, physiotherapists, psychologists, and social workers. As a model treatment program, CVT has provided services to more than 500 survivors and their family members from more than 50 countries of origin. More than half of those treated are from Africa, with significant numbers from Southeast Asia and Latin America, smaller numbers from the Middle East and Eastern

Europe, and a few U.S. citizens who were tortured abroad. Eighty percent of CVT's resources are allocated to survivors living in Minnesota at the time treatment is sought; 20% are reserved for those who travel to Minnesota for treatment. In recent years, as a result of the availability of other centers in the United States, the vast majority of survivors treated at CVT are persons living in Minnesota.

By 1990, the caseload at CVT had increased to neary 150 new and ongoing clients annually, most provided with free outpatient care. Even at this rate of service provision, it would take CVT nearly 50 years to provide direct care to only the estimated 12,000 survivors already living in Minnesota. As a result, the board of directors decided to limit to 120 the number of clients treated per year and to shift the focus to initiatives that would enable the organization to serve larger numbers of people and to serve as a source of learning for others, who would in turn find new ways of caring for torture survivors.

This shift in CVT's direction provided the opportunity to initiate projects in the former Yugoslavia. After the AID fact-finding mission in February 1993, CVT organized a training and assessment team, which visited Croatia in April 1993. The team consisted of CVT's international training coordinator (a nurse and public health specialist by background), a family practitioner, and a psychologist. The team's objectives were 1) to assess the long-term training and support needs in the region; 2) to conduct training for agencies or individuals who provide assistance to traumatized refugees; and 3) to understand the range of experiences of trauma survivors in the former Yugoslavia, in an attempt to influence clinical activities and training efforts in areas where survivors are resettled.

On its return, the team recommended that CVT take an increasingly active role in the former Yugoslavia and focus its efforts on training and program development. Shortly thereafter, AID requested that CVT conduct a training program in Minneapolis for health care professionals from Bosnia and Croatia. In November 1993, CVT hosted a group of 14 service providers, both professionals and paraprofessionals, for an intensive 3½-week training session focusing on clinical issues related to torture, rape, and war trauma, as well as on program development and capacity-building initiatives. Major goals were not only to improve the clinical skills of the participants but also to increase participants' levels of confidence. Special issues in the curriculum included the treatment of former prisoners of war, veterans, and victims of sexual torture and the impact of war and violence on children and families. At the request of the participants, an extra session was added, in which participants developed a strategic plan for CVT's presence in Croatia and Bosnia. This activity helped to demonstrate the steps involved in the process and to determine an appropriate role for CVT in the region.

In addition, the risks of retraumatization in the victims and "vicarious traumatization" in the caregivers were addressed. One of the participants from Bosnia shared her experience of being distressed whenever one of her clients was late for a therapy appointment; this distress came from fearing the client had been killed attempting to cross a bridge en route to the office. During the training in Minnesota, several participants were moved to tears in a field visit to a program treating sexually assaulted children. This may have been a type of delayed vicarious traumatization; they had certainly seen far worse evidence and heard far worse accounts of sexual assault on children in their own country.

CVT's mental health professionals had anticipated a need for intervention in cases of reactions such as these, and therefore group debriefing sessions were provided in the evenings. In addition, formal presentations on vicarious traumatization were given earlier in the training and were integrated into the entire curriculum. Although it was not a written goal of the training program, development of a strong group process and group communication occurred. The participants were very satisfied with the development of this group process, which increased trust among this diverse group of former Yugoslavians and coincided well with the training philosophy of CVT. The project received extremely positive evaluations not only from the participants, but also from the AID representative monitoring the project (C. Robertson, unpublished report, December 1993). A second training program, with 12 participants, was subsequently conducted. In designing this program, CVT took into account feedback from the first training program. The content of the second program was similar to that of the first, but the second program was shorter and had fewer didactic sessions, greater interaction in the form of intimate group discussions, and a smaller number of field groups.

During the initial training program, representatives of virtually every participating organization requested partnership with CVT on site in the former Yugoslavia. The consensus was that there was a need for intensive capacity building and training in organizational development, volunteer management, and program evaluation on site.

Subsequently, CVT sent its training contractor to Croatia and Bosnia to take care of the very complicated logistics of providing a training program in the former Yugoslavia. The CVT then sent a team—consisting of a psychologist, the volunteer coordinator from CVT, and the volunteer coordinator from the Canadian Centre for Victims of Torture in Toronto— to Croatia for a 2-week period to consult primarily with Merhamet, one of the local organizations, but with others as well. The team offered strategies for dealing with vicarious traumatization among the on-site professional staff and volunteers and assisted in the development, management, and coordination of volunteers. This short initial training mission laid the groundwork for the subsequent 4-month stay in Croatia by the team's psychologist, who assisted with capacity building, training, and provision of direct services to caregivers and clients. This approach fit well with CVT's new priorities, given that tens of thousands of torture survivors will want and need to remain in Croatia and Bosnia.

Conclusion

Treatment strategies are most effective when they involve local sources of social, cultural, and organizational support. Many of the agencies now working in the former Yugoslavia admit to a lack of knowledge in the specialized practice of treating torture survivors. The training these agencies request clearly must be given in the communities they serve. The organizations must also plan to serve victims until long after the violence in the former Yugoslavia ends, because it is very possible that the need for psychological rehabilitation and recovery will be even greater when the atrocities cease.

Ultimately, stopping the violence of war and torture would help significantly in preventing the epidemic of posttraumatic stress disorders that plague the millions of refugees and displaced persons worldwide. In the meantime, rushing to the scene with only the tools to treat the bodily injuries is not enough. Later, when the broken bones have healed, it is the nightmares that haunt refugees. Sound psychological interventions employed as soon as possible could go a long way in promoting recovery and fostering the building of new lives out of profound tragedy.

References

Anthony CR, Witterholt SW, Boothby N, et al: Assistance for victims of atrocities in Croatia and Bosnia-Herzegovina. Washington, DC, U.S. Agency for International Development, 1993

Arcel LT, Folnegovic-Smale V, Kozaric-Kovacic D, et al. (eds): Psycho-Social Help to War Victims: Women Refugees and Their Families. Copenhagen, International Rehabilitation Council for Torture Victims, 1995

Camp NM: The Vietnam War and the ethics of combat psychiatry. Am J Psychiatry 150:1000–1010, 1993

Chester B: Because mercy has a human heart: centers for victims of torture, in Psychology and Torture. Edited by Suedfeld P. Washington, DC, Hemisphere, 1990, pp 165–184

Fletcher L, Musalo K, Urentlicher D, et al: No Justice, No Peace: Accountability for Rape and Gender-Based Violence in the Former Yugoslavia. Washington, DC, International Human Rights Law Group, 1993

Garcia-Peltoniemi RE, Jaranson J: A multidisciplinary approach to the treatment of torture victims. Abstract of paper presented at the 2nd International Conference of Centres, Institutions and Individuals Concerned With the Care of Victims of Organized Violence. San José, Costa Rica, November 27–December 2, 1989

Loveridge D: Report on visit to Bosnia and Croatia for the period April 8, 1993–June 19, 1993. IRC Mental Health Programme, June 18, 1993

McCann L, Pearlman LA: Vicarious traumatization: a framework for understanding the psychological effects of working with victims. J Trauma Stress 3:131–148, 1990

Riding A: European inquiry says Serbs' forces raped 20,000. The New York Times, January 9, 1993, pp 1, 4

U.S. Agency for International Development: Situation Report No. 8. Washington, DC, U.S. Agency for International Development, 1993, pp 1–10

World Conference on Human Rights, Women's Commission of Refugee Women and Children: Violence against refugee and displaced women and children—findings and remedies. Paper presented at World Conference on Human Rights, June 1993

Index

Page numbers printed in boldface type refer to tables or figures.